Cancer Rehabilitation

Jennifer Baima · Ashish Khanna
Editors

Cancer Rehabilitation

A Concise and Portable Pocket Guide

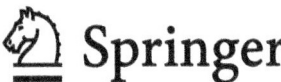 Springer

Editors
Jennifer Baima
Orthopedics and Physical
Rehabilitation
University of Massachusetts
Medical School
Worcester, MA
USA

Ashish Khanna
Physical Medicine
and Rehabilitation
Rutgers New Jersey
Medical School
The Kessler Institute
for Rehabilitation
West Orange, NY
USA

ISBN 978-3-030-44461-7   ISBN 978-3-030-44462-4 (eBook)
https://doi.org/10.1007/978-3-030-44462-4

This Springer imprint is published by the registered company Springer Nature Switzerland AG
The registered company address is: Gewerbestrasse 11, 6330 Cham, Switzerland

Acknowledgments

We would like to thank all of the past, current, and future members of the Cancer Rehabilitation Physicians Consortium (CRPC) who have worked tirelessly to improve access to cancer rehabilitation medicine for our patients.

Jennifer Baima

I would like to dedicate this book to my parents, Alka and Ashok, who epitomize the qualities of great physicians and "strongly encouraged" me to also become one (you were right); to my wife, Meghan, without whose superior intellect, love, and example through medical school and training I would have never made it; to my ever-inspiring superhero-in-a-small-package sister, Ashima; to my mentors, Drs. Adrian Cristian and Eric Wisotzky, who believed in me for whatever reason; and lastly, to my son, Daksh, born during the writing of this book, without whom it would have been completed much earlier.

Ashish Khanna

Contents

Contributors

Alba Azola Department of Physical Medicine and Rehabilitation, Johns Hopkins University School of Medicine, Baltimore, MD, USA

Andrea Cheville Department of Physical Medicine and Rehabilitation, Mayo Clinic, Rochester, MN, USA

Kathy Chou Physical Medicine and Rehabilitation, Kessler Institute for Rehabilitation, West Orange, NJ, USA

Nabela Enam Physical Medicine and Rehabilitation, Kessler Institute for Rehabilitation, West Orange, NJ, USA

Michael Fediw University of Michigan, Department of Physical Medicine and Rehabilitation, Ann Arbor, MI, USA

George Francis Physical Medicine and Rehabilitation, Tom Baker Cancer Center, University of Calgary, Calgary, AB, Canada

Ekta Gupta Department of Palliative, Rehabilitation and Integrative Medicine, University of Texas MD Anderson Cancer Center, Houston, TX, USA

John Haskoor Department of Orthopedics and Physical Rehabilitation, University of Massachusetts Medical School, Worcester, MA, USA

Ashish Khanna Physical Medicine and Rehabilitation, Rutgers New Jersey Medical School, The Kessler Institute for Rehabilitation, West Orange, NY, USA

R. Samuel Mayer Department of Physical Medicine and Rehabilitation, Johns Hopkins University School of Medicine, Baltimore, MD, USA

Charles Mitchell Oncology Rehabilitation at Carolinas Rehabilitation of Atrium Health, Charlotte, NC, USA

Cancer Rehabilitation Section of Rehabilitation Department of Supportive Care at Levine Cancer Institute, Charlotte, NC, USA

Diana Molinares Department of Palliative, Rehabilitation and Integrative Medicine, University of Texas MD Anderson Cancer Center, Houston, TX, USA

Mathew J. Most Division of Orthopedic Oncology, Department of Orthopedics and Physical Rehabilitation, UMass Memorial HealthCare, Worcester, MA, USA

An Ngo-Huang Palliative, Rehabilitation, and Integrative Medicine, University of Texas MD Anderson Cancer Center, Houston, TX, USA

Sara Parke Department of Palliative, Rehabilitation and Integrative Medicine, University of Texas MD Anderson Cancer Center, Houston, TX, USA

Katherine Power MedStar National Rehabilitation Hospital, Physical Medicine and Rehabilitation, Washington, DC, USA

Terrence Pugh Oncology Rehabilitation at Carolinas Rehabilitation of Atrium Health, Charlotte, NC, USA

Cancer Rehabilitation Section of Rehabilitation Department of Supportive Care at Levine Cancer Institute, Charlotte, NC, USA

Vishwa Raj Oncology Rehabilitation at Carolinas Rehabilitation of Atrium Health, Charlotte, NC, USA

Cancer Rehabilitation Section of Rehabilitation Department of Supportive Care at Levine Cancer Institute, Charlotte, NC, USA

Julie K. Silver Department of Physical Medicine and Rehabilitation, Harvard Medical School, Boston, MA, USA

Spaulding Rehabilitation Hospital, Boston, MA, USA

Massachusetts General Hospital, Boston, MA, USA

Brigham and Women's Hospital, Boston, MA, USA

Sean Smith University of Michigan, Department of Physical Medicine and Rehabilitation, Ann Arbor, MI, USA

Michael Stubblefield Physical Medicine and Rehabilitation, Kessler Institute for Rehabilitation, West Orange, NJ, USA

Grigory Syrkin Department of Neurology, Rehabilitation Medicine Service, Memorial Sloan Kettering Cancer Center, New York, NY, USA

Mary Vargo Metro Health Medical Center, Department of Physical Medicine and Rehabilitation, Case Western Reserve University, Cleveland, OH, USA

Chapter 1
Integrating Impairment-Driven Cancer Rehabilitation into the Care Continuum

Julie K. Silver

Cancer is one of the most common, disabling, and costly diagnoses that affects people living in the USA and worldwide. Today, nearly 40% of people will develop cancer in their lifetime [1]. Due to many advances in oncology therapies, the overall 5-year survival rate has steadily increased and is currently hovering around 67% [1]. As a result, there are more than 15.5 million cancer survivors living in the USA [2], and by 2020, the US Centers for Disease Control and Prevention (CDC) projects there will be more than 18 million Americans living with cancer [3].

However, even though there is an increase in the overall 5-year survival rate, survival is not necessarily disease free, and often people live with cancer as a chronic condition. Although many people with advanced cancer will ultimately

J. K. Silver (✉)
Department of Physical Medicine and Rehabilitation, Harvard Medical School, Boston, MA, USA

Spaulding Rehabilitation Hospital, Boston, MA, USA

Massachusetts General Hospital, Boston, MA, USA

Brigham and Women's Hospital, Boston, MA, USA
e-mail: julie_silver@hms.harvard.edu

© Springer Nature Switzerland AG 2020
J. Baima, A. Khanna (eds.), *Cancer Rehabilitation*,
https://doi.org/10.1007/978-3-030-44462-4_1

succumb to complications related to progression of their malignancy, increasingly, an oncological diagnosis may not be the cause of mortality. Nearly everyone who lives with cancer as a chronic condition will experience significant and progressive morbidity and functional disability over time. This is in large part because they are subjected to a combination of oncology-directed therapies (e.g., surgery, chemotherapy, and/or radiation therapy) that are often delivered sequentially or even simultaneously over months or years. The cumulative effect of cancer and/or its treatment increases the functional morbidity burden. Newer therapies, such as targeted treatments, may further increase survival rates while at the same time contribute to more morbidity and disability for survivors. Therefore, there is a growing need for cancer rehabilitation.

The Rise of Cancer Rehabilitation

Historically, cancer rehabilitation was not well integrated into oncology care. Although programs were described in the late 1960s and 1970s when research began to demonstrate the efficacy of interventions [4, 5], they generally focused on specific patient populations (e.g., breast cancer survivors or problems such as lymphedema). More recently research has demonstrated that cancer survivors may have multiple impairments that are not treated [6–8]. Not surprisingly, studies have also shown a link between physical and functional problems in survivors and psychological sequelae [9–12]. Unfortunately, this means that many patients are experiencing *unnecessary* physical and psychological suffering [13]. Indeed, while the field of cancer rehabilitation has been present for decades, it has grown a lot recently, and there is an urgent need to diagnose and treat the many impairments that cancer or its treatments may cause. In fact, there is an urgent need to integrate *impairment-driven cancer rehabilitation* into the care continuum. Impairments come in many forms and may affect any organ system in the body (Table 1.1). Moreover, because of the nature of oncologic-directed therapies that occur sequentially or simultaneously, patients tend to acquire multiple impairments, and these often become cumulative over time.

TABLE 1.1 Examples of impairments in cancer survivors

Head and neck cancer: pain, weakness, endurance, fatigue, swallowing, cervical and shoulder range of motion

Prostate Cancer: pain, weakness, endurance, fatigue, urinary and erectile dysfunction

Breast Cancer: pain, weakness, endurance, fatigue, neuropathy, lymphedema, upper quadrant morbidity

Leukemia: pain, weakness, endurance, fatigue, graft versus host disease

Legend: These are examples of the types of symptoms and impairments that cancer patients may have. This is not intended to be a complete list of cancers or impairments

For rehabilitation specialists, it is crucial to educate colleagues and patients about cancer rehabilitation care as we know from the literature that there is a tremendous lack of knowledge. For example, one report published in an oncology journal was titled, "I didn't actually know there was such a thing as rehab: Survivor, family, and clinician perceptions of rehabilitation following treatment for head and neck cancer" and highlighted patients' confusion about crucial services that they would benefit from [14]. The author of this chapter led a study which found that more than 90% of National Cancer Institute (NCI)-designated cancer centers that provide clinical care did not have an easily identifiable patient-focused description of or link to cancer rehabilitation services on their website and that only 8% of the websites included accurate and detailed information that referenced four core rehabilitation services (physiatry and physical, occupational, and speech therapy) [15].

Definition of Cancer Rehabilitation

"Cancer rehabilitation is medical care that should be integrated throughout the oncology care continuum and delivered by trained rehabilitation professionals who have it within their scope of practice to diagnose and treat patients' physical, cognitive and functional impairments in an effort to maintain or restore function, reduce symptom burden, maximize independence and improve quality of life in this medically complex population."

Silver et al. [16].

Successful integration of cancer rehabilitation will require developing the workforce to care for the many patients who need this care. Screening patients who are newly diagnosed and throughout active cancer treatment and survivorship is important. The prospective surveillance model has been proposed as one way to do this [17].

On the oncology side, there has been a growing emphasis on survivorship care, which has provided an opportunity for cancer rehabilitation to become better integrated into the oncology care continuum. For example, a series of reports published by the Institute of Medicine has prompted both discussion and action regarding establishing survivorship as a distinct component of oncology care. The report "From Cancer Patient to Cancer Survivor: Lost in Transition," explained how people are often left with long-term pain, fatigue and other physical and functional problems after their malignancy is treated [18]. The report, "Cancer Care for the Whole Patient: Meeting Psychosocial Health Needs," highlighted the psychosocial sequelae in survivors [19]. The report, "Delivering High-Quality Cancer Care," suggested a now adopted framework for patient-centered care that involved quality metrics and new payment models [20]. These reports encouraged oncology specialists to focus on survival as well as other metrics that involve physical and emotional functioning, and quality of life outcomes.

Notably, exercise is one important component of helping survivors regain their strength and endurance and has a strong evidence base [21]; however, individuals tend to have numerous other impairments that may affect nearly every system in the body. For example, people who have been treated for head and neck cancer may experience impairments with speech, swallowing, cervical range of motion, peripheral neuropathy, etc. Those who are diagnosed with brain or spinal cord tumors may have complex rehabilitation needs similar to people who have had a stroke, traumatic brain or spinal cord injury.

Therefore, they may benefit from a well-coordinated interdisciplinary rehabilitation services approach.

Following the aforementioned reports and other published studies, one important cancer rehabilitation initiative that began in 2015 and was led by the Rehabilitation Medicine Department at the National Institutes of Health (NIH) with support from the NCI and the National Center for Medical Rehabilitation Research convened a group of subject matter experts to review the current evidence base and practice patterns. The goal was to identify opportunities for research and enhanced clinical integration, and the group produced a report with 10 specific recommendations aimed at achieving this goal by helping stakeholders identify the most important areas to focus on to advance the field (Table 1.2) [22]. It is

TABLE 1.2 Cancer rehabilitation integration recommendations

1.	Provide rehabilitation screening
2.	Incorporate objective assessment of functional status
3.	Utilize national reports to guide survivorship care
4.	Offer prehabilitation when appropriate
5.	Assess current clinical tools and metrics
6.	Create a centralized electronic interface to facilitate data collection
7.	Develop practice guidelines
8.	Expand education and training
9.	Elevate awareness
10.	Identify research gaps

Legend: These recommendations are adapted from the cancer rehabilitation initiative that began in 2015 and was led by the Rehabilitation Medicine Department at the National Institutes of Health with support from the National Cancer Institute and the National Center for Medical Rehabilitation Research
Ref: Stout NL, Silver JK, Raj VS, et al. Toward a National Initiative in Cancer Rehabilitation: Recommendations From a Subject Matter Expert Group. *Arch Phys Med Rehabil.* 2016;97(11):2006–2015

essential to emphasize the role of the physiatrist [23], safety concerns in these complicated patients [24, 25], and employment and disability issues [26, 27]. These important topics will be covered throughout this book.

The Rise of Cancer Prehabilitation

Prehabilitation has been utilized in the care of patients with varied diagnoses, including but not limited to orthopedics, and it is increasingly an important part of cancer rehabilitation care. The basic concept behind all prehabilitation is aimed at preparing someone for an upcoming stressor such as surgery.

Definition of Cancer Prehabilitation

"Prehabilitation is a process on the cancer continuum of care that occurs between the time of cancer diagnosis and the beginning of acute treatment and includes physical and psychological assessments that establish a baseline functional level, identify impairments, and provide interventions that promote physical and psychological health to reduce the incidence and/or severity of future impairments."

Silver et al. [13].

Since the first review was published on the topic of cancer prehabilitation, the field has grown [28]. For example, in 2015, a group of subject matter experts in surgical cancer prehabilitation convened in Canada to reach consensus regarding recommendations for future research [29]. Prehabilitation is evolving in an effort to improve the physical, emotional, and functional outcomes as well as to positively affect adherence to adjuvant treatment, value-based care, and even survival (Table 1.3) [30, 31].

Prehabilitation is often best delivered in a multimodal approach, rather than as a single modality such as exercise only [29]. For example, one breast cancer prehabilitation protocol described exercise to build endurance and strength, nutrition with protein supplementation, stress reduction tech-

TABLE 1.3 Potential goals and benefits of cancer prehabilitation

Improved physical, cognitive, psychological, and functional outcomes

Increased adherence to cancer-directed therapy (e.g., chemotherapy)

Reduced complications (e.g., post-surgical respiratory problems)

Decreased risk of hospital readmissions or emergency department visits

Legend: Prehabilitation interventions may support a variety of health outcomes. This is not intended to be a complete list

Prehabilitation	Peri-operative enhanced recovery programs	Rehabilitation
Diagnosis	Surgery	Post-op

FIGURE 1.1 Integrating cancer prehabilitation and rehabilitation into the surgical care continuum. Legend: Cancer prehabilitation often begins shortly after diagnosis. Perioperative early recovery programs are usually administered in the 48–72 hours before, during, and after surgery and this is followed by conventional rehabilitation

niques, and smoking cessation [31]. A similar approach was suggested for patients with lung cancer, particularly with the adoption of low-dose computed tomography (CT) screening that is aimed at identifying tumors at an earlier stage whereby they may be surgically resectable and patients are treated with curative intent [32].

Prehabilitation fits into the care continuum shortly after diagnosis, and for those patients who will be undergoing surgery, this may be integrated with perioperative early recovery programs that have been well documented in the literature to be effective in supporting positive outcomes (Fig. 1.1).

The Rise of Palliative Care

Cancer rehabilitation and palliative care often intersect and providers in both specialty areas can facilitate appropriate referrals that support well-integrated care and optimal outcomes for patients [16].

Definition of Palliative Care

"Palliative care is specialized medical care for people with serious illnesses. This type of care is focused on providing patients with relief from the symptoms, pain and stress of a serious illness—whatever the diagnosis. The goal is to improve quality of life for both the patient and the family. Palliative care is provided by a team of doctors, nurses, and other specialists who work with a patient's other doctors to provide an extra layer of support. Palliative care is appropriate at any age and at any state in a serious illness, and can be provided together with curative treatment."

Center to Advance Palliative Care [33].

Palliative care has undergone a transformation that has provided a pathway toward the growth of the field. A recent report explained the changes and suggested that the field of cancer rehabilitation might benefit from a similar approach [34]. The report suggested a strategic approach by:

1. Stimulating the science in specific gap areas
2. Creating clinical practice guidelines
3. Building clinical capacity
4. Ascertaining and responding to public opinion
5. Advocating for public policy change

This report provides a path forward for the field of cancer rehabilitation and the integration of these services into the care continuum.

Cancer prehabilitation and rehabilitation are important components of oncology care and help to optimize patients' physical, psychological, and functional outcomes, regardless of whether they are cured or live with cancer as a chronic condition.

Disclosure of Funding   None.

References

1. Surveillance Epidemiology and End Results [SEER] Program cancer stat facts: cancer of any site. National Cancer Institute.

Available at: https://seer.cancer.gov/statfacts/html/all.html. Accessed 23 July 2017.

2. American Cancer Society. Cancer facts & figures 2017. Atlanta: American Cancer Society; 2017.

3. Expected new cancer cases and deaths in 2020. US Department of Health & Human Services Centers for Disease Control and Prevention. Available at: https://www.cdc.gov/cancer/dcpc/research/articles/cancer_2020.htm. Published 2016. Accessed 23 July 2017.

4. Dietz JH Jr. Rehabilitation of the cancer patient. Med Clin North Am. 1969;53(3):607–24.

5. Lehmann JF, DeLisa JA, Warren CG, de Lateur BJ, Bryant PL, Nicholson CG. Cancer rehabilitation: assessment of need, development, and evaluation of a model of care. Arch Phys Med Rehabil. 1978;59(9):410–9.

6. Cheville AL, Troxel AB, Basford JR, Kornblith AB. Prevalence and treatment patterns of physical impairments in patients with metastatic breast cancer. J Clin Oncol. 2008;26(16):2621–9.

7. Cheville AL, Beck LA, Petersen TL, Marks RS, Gamble GL. The detection and treatment of cancer-related functional problems in an outpatient setting. Support Care Cancer. 2009;17(1):61–7.

8. Pergolotti M, Deal AM, Lavery J, Reeve BB, Muss HB. The prevalence of potentially modifiable functional deficits and the subsequent use of occupational and physical therapy by older adults with cancer. J Geriatr Oncol. 2015;6(3):194–201.

9. Bevans MF, Mitchell SA, Barrett JA, et al. Symptom distress predicts long-term health and well-being in allogeneic stem cell transplantation survivors. Biol Blood Marrow Transplant. 2014;20(3):387–95.

10. Penttinen HM, Saarto T, Kellokumpu-Lehtinen P, et al. Quality of life and physical performance and activity of breast cancer patients after adjuvant treatments. Psychooncology. 2011;20(11):1211–20.

11. Banks E, Byles JE, Gibson RE, et al. Is psychological distress in people living with cancer related to the fact of diagnosis, current treatment or level of disability? Findings from a large Australian study. Med J Aust. 2010;193(5 Suppl):S62–7.

12. Weaver KE, Forsythe LP, Reeve BB, et al. Mental and physical health-related quality of life among U.S. cancer survivors: population estimates from the 2010 National Health Interview Survey. Cancer Epidemiol Biomark Prev. 2012;21(11):2108–17.

13. Silver JK, Baima J, Mayer RS. Impairment-driven cancer rehabilitation: an essential component of quality care and survivorship. CA Cancer J Clin. 2013;63(5):295–317.

14. McEwen S, Rodriguez AM, Martino R, Poon I, Dunphy C, Rios JN, Ringash J. "I didn't actually know there was such a thing as rehab": survivor, family, and clinician perceptions of rehabilitation following treatment for head and neck cancer. Support Care Cancer. 2016;24(4):1449–53.
15. Silver JK, Raj VS, Fu JB, et al. Most National Cancer Institute-designated cancer center websites do not provide survivors with information about cancer rehabilitation services. J Cancer Educ. 2018;33(5):947–53.
16. Silver JK, Raj VS, Fu JB, Wisotzky EM, Smith SR, Kirch RA. Cancer rehabilitation and palliative care: critical components in the delivery of high-quality oncology care services. Support Care Cancer. 2015;23:3633–43.
17. Stout NL, Silver JK, Alfano CM, Ness KK, Gilchrist LS. Long-term survivorship care after cancer treatment: a new emphasis on the role of rehabilitation services. Phys Ther. 2019;99(1):10–3.
18. Institute of Medicine, National Research Council. From cancer patient to cancer survivor: lost in transition. Washington, DC: National Academies Press; 2005.
19. Institute of Medicine. Cancer care for the whole patient: meeting psychosocial health needs. Washington, DC: The National Academies Press; 2008.
20. Institute of Medicine. Delivering high-quality cancer care: charting a new course for a system in crisis. Washington, DC: National Academies Press; 2013.
21. Stout NL, Baima J, Swisher A, et al. A systematic review of exercise systematic reviews in the cancer literature (2005-2017). PM R. 2017;9(9S2):S347–84.
22. Stout NL, Silver JK, Raj VS, et al. Toward a national initiative in cancer rehabilitation: recommendations from a subject matter expert group. Arch Phys Med Rehabil. 2016;97(11):2006–15.
23. Smith SR, Reish AG, Andrews C. Cancer survivorship: a growing role for physiatric care. PM R. 2015;7(5):527–31. https://doi.org/10.1016/j.pmrj.2014.12.004.
24. Cristian A, Tran A, Patel K. Patient safety in cancer rehabilitation. Phys Med Rehabil Clin N Am. 2012;23(2):441–56. https://doi.org/10.1016/j.pmr.2012.02.015.
25. Maltser S, Cristian A, Silver JK, et al. A focused review of safety considerations in cancer rehabilitation. PM R. 2017;9(9S2):S415–28.
26. Silver JK, Baima J, Newman R, Galantino ML, Shockney LD. Cancer rehabilitation may improve function in survivors

and decrease the economic burden of cancer to society. Work. 2013;46:455–72.

27. Alfano CM, Kent EE, Padgett LS, et al. Making cancer rehabilitation services work for cancer patients: recommendations for research and practice to improve employment outcomes. PM R. 2017;9(9S2):S398–406.

28. Silver JK, Baima J. Cancer prehabilitation: an opportunity to decrease treatment-related morbidity, increase cancer treatment options and improve physical and psychological health outcomes. Am J Phys Med Rehabil. 2013;92(8):715–27.

29. Carli F, Silver JK, Feldman LS, et al. Surgical prehabilitation in patients with cancer: state-of-the-science and recommendations for future research from a panel of subject matter experts. Phys Med Rehabil Clin N Am. 2017;28(1):49–64.

30. Smith SR, Khanna A, Wisotzky EM. An evolving role for cancer rehabilitation in the era of low dose lung CT screening. PM R. 2017;9(9S2):S407–14.

31. Santa Mina D, Brahmbhatt P, Lopez C, et al. The case for prehabilitation prior to breast cancer treatment. PM R. 2017;9(9S2):S305–16.

32. Smith SR, Khanna A, Wisotzky EM. An evolving role for cancer rehabilitation in the era of low-dose lung computed tomography screening. PM R. 2017;9(9S2):S407–14.

33. Center to Advance Palliative Care (2011) Public opinion research on palliative care. https://media.capc.org/filer_public/18/ab/18ab708c-f835-4380-921d-fbf729702e36/2011-public-opinion-research-on-palliative-care.pdf. Accessed 7 Feb 2019

34. Lyons KD, Padgett LS, Marshall TF, et al. Follow the trail: using insight from the growth of palliative care to propose a roadmap for cancer rehabilitation. CA Cancer J Clin. 2018; https://doi.org/10.3322/caac.21549. [Epub ahead of print].

Chapter 2
Breast Cancer Rehabilitation

Katherine Power and Ashish Khanna

Breast cancer is the most commonly diagnosed cancer among women in the USA and it has a five-year survival rate of nearly 90% [1]. Consequentially, millions of breast cancer survivors are living with the effects of their cancer and its treatment. There are several pathological types of breast cancer; the most common is invasive intraductal carcinoma. The oncological treatment plan will vary slightly based on this pathology, but will often include surgery, chemotherapy, radiation, and/or endocrine therapy. Surgery may involve a lumpectomy which preserves the remaining breast tissue after excision with adequate margins, or mastectomy which involves removal of all the breast tissue (with or without skin and nipple). Often a sentinel lymph node biopsy (SLNB) is done in the axilla on the affected side, which entails removal of one or a few lymph nodes. Sometimes an axillary lymph node dissection (ALND) is performed, which entails removal of several lymph nodes

K. Power (✉)
MedStar National Rehabilitation Hospital, Physical Medicine and Rehabilitation, Washington, DC, USA
e-mail: Katherine.x.power@medstar.net

A. Khanna
Physical Medicine and Rehabilitation,
Rutgers New Jersey Medical School,
The Kessler Institute for Rehabilitation, West Orange, NY, USA

© Springer Nature Switzerland AG 2020
J. Baima, A. Khanna (eds.), *Cancer Rehabilitation*,
https://doi.org/10.1007/978-3-030-44462-4_2

typically located in levels I and II of axilla [2]. In addition, many women opt for breast reconstruction surgery which may be done at the time of their original surgery or at later date. Chemotherapy is part of the treatment plan for many breast cancer patients and can be administered in a neo-adjuvant setting or given as adjuvant therapy. Radiation is typically performed after the patient has undergone surgery. Hormone therapy is given to certain breast cancer survivors to reduce risk of recurrence. These medications are taken daily for 5–10 years [3]. Tamoxifen is typically given to pre-menopausal patients, and aromatase inhibitors (anastrozole, letrozole, and exemestane) are given to postmenopausal women.

There are certain characteristics of the cancer that will affect a patient's outcome and the possibility of developing impairments. First, the hormone receptor status has an effect. When patients undergo breast biopsy, the sample will be tested for estrogen receptor (ER) and progesterone receptor (PR) expression. About 60–75% of all breast cancer cases can be classified as estrogen receptor positive [4]. Similarly, the HER2 (human epidermal growth receptor 2) status is determined. When one is negative for ER, PR, and HER2 expression they are said to be 'triple negative.' Triple negative breast cancers have a lower five-year survival rate. Another important factor is the presence of local or distal metastases. Local cancer spread refers to presence of cancer in axillary lymph nodes. The prognosis is least favorable for patients with distant metastases. Common sites of distant metastases for breast cancer include bone, lung, liver, and brain [5].

Impairments

From the time of the diagnosis of breast cancer and throughout the entirety of a survivors' life, there are several impairments that can develop. Some can be directly related to the presence of the tumor itself and others are related to the medical and surgical treatments of that cancer. Table 2.1

TABLE 2.1 Summary of common impairments in breast cancer

Impairment	Typical onset	Possible etiology	Clinical	Prognosis
Postmastectomy pain syndrome	After any breast surgery	Nerve damage, incisional pain, altered biomechanics, myofascial pain	Pain in chest wall, axilla, or upper arm, limited shoulder Range of motion (ROM)	With treatment will often improve
Peripheral neuropathy	During or shortly after chemotherapy	Toxic effect of chemotherapy agents on nerves	Paresthesias in feet > hands, fine motor issues, imbalance	May improve with more time since exposure or persist
Lymphedema	Months to years after lymph node removal	Iatrogenic node resection impairing lymph flow or pathologic lymph node	Edematous limb, heaviness of limb, increased risk of infections	Non-curative but can be improved
Radiation fibrosis	Months to years	Tissue damage involving chest wall due to radiation exposure	Limited shoulder ROM, chest wall pain	With treatment will often improve, without can worsen

(continued)

TABLE 2.1 (continued)

Impairment	Typical onset	Possible etiology	Clinical	Prognosis
Aromatase-inhibitor-associated musculoskeletal symptoms	Weeks to months after starting an aromatase inhibitor	Not fully understood	Localized or diffuse joint pain and/or muscle pain	With treatment can improve
Fatigue	At time of diagnosis or during any stage of treatment	May involve tumor itself, chemotherapy, or radiation	Lack of energy, endurance	With time and/or treatment should improve
Cancer-associated cognitive dysfunction	At time of diagnosis or during any stage of treatment	May involve tumor itself, chemotherapy, radiation, or endocrine therapy	Memory impairment, trouble focusing, poor attention	With time and/or treatment can improve
Brachial plexopathy	Several years after radiation or when tumor develops locally	Radiation exposure to plexus or direct tumor effect	Weakness of affected Upper extremity (UE), pain in affected UE	If due to radiation it is slowly progressive, if due to tumor, more rapidly progressive

shows some of the common impairments, when they typically occur, and possible etiologies. Those more common to breast cancer than other cancer types are discussed below.

Postmastectomy pain syndrome (PMPS) involves persistent pain, typically more than 3 months, following any breast surgery [6]. Pain can be located in the chest wall, axilla, arm, or shoulder on the affected side. Range of motion issues typically accompany the pain. Several studies have looked at what attributes increases a patient's risk for development of PMPS. The incidence of PMPS has been shown to be higher in patients with higher severity of acute postoperative pain, those who undergo axillary lymph node dissections, and those who receive radiation [7]. Interestingly, one paper reported no specific treatment increased one's risk of developing PMPS; instead poor psychological coping tactics such as catastrophizing was the most significant risk factor for PMPS development [8].

It can be helpful to think of PMPS as a constellation of individual diagnoses such as: intercostobrachial neuralgia, incisional pain, cording, or shoulder dysfunction. It can also involve more than one of these diagnoses at a time. Intercostobrachial neuralgia can develop due to direct damage or partial transection during surgery or due to compression from surrounding scar tissue. Patients often describe either numbness or paresthesias in the distribution of the intercostobrachial nerve (lateral chest wall, axilla, medial upper arm). Neuropathic pain medications have been used to treat these paresthesias but there have not been a lot of research to support use of one over another [7]. Cording, also known as axillary web syndrome, is thought to be caused by sclerosis or thrombosis of the axillary veins and/or lymphatics. This will often result in reduced shoulder range of motion. It is typically self-limiting, but the discomfort and reduced ROM can be improved more rapidly with manual therapy techniques in physical therapy [9].

Both rotator cuff syndrome and adhesive capsulitis can develop postoperatively in these patients. The higher incidence is thought to be due to the change in biomechanics that

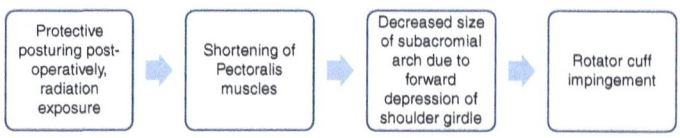

FIGURE 2.1 Biomechanical changes in the shoulder following breast cancer treatments

occurs following surgery [10]. These changes are depicted in Fig. 2.1 below. Treatment for both rotator cuff syndrome and adhesive capsulitis is typically the same as in the noncancer population (physical therapy, anti-inflammatories, corticosteroid injections, percutaneous tenotomy). Knowing that these patients are at higher risk for developing these conditions can help providers educate patients on trying to maintain their ROM prior to surgery and as allowed by their surgeon in the postoperative period.

Aromatase-inhibitor-induced musculoskeletal symptoms (AIMSS) classically consist of arthralgias and tendinopathies. The pathophysiology behind their development is not fully understood. As a group, they are among the most common side effects associated with use of AIs, with studies reporting incidence as high as 50–82% [11, 12]. These symptoms typically develop within the first several weeks of starting an AI [13]. Arthralgias can affect any part of the body but the most common areas that patients report them in are wrists/hands followed by knees. De Quervain's tenosynovitis, trigger fingers, and carpal tunnel syndrome are often seen. Interestingly, carpal tunnel syndrome is thought to develop secondary to AI usage because of tenosynovitis of the tendons in the carpal tunnel.

Because of the differences in presentation there is no one accepted treatment strategy for AIMSS. One proposed approach is to first determine if patient is having only focal symptoms, or more diffuse symptoms [14]. For example, if patient develops symptoms of De Quervain's tenosynovitis after starting an AI, the treatment plan would be the same as if they had it without use of an AI. This might include NSAIDs, splinting, hand therapy, and/or corticosteroid injection. If symptoms are more widespread, the strategy changes. Several studies have looked at different treatments for AIMSS. Regular moderate-intensity exercise involving strengthening and aerobic activity has been shown to decrease pain scores [15]. Smaller studies have looked at specific exercise types such as yoga, aquatic therapy, tai chi, and walking. No specific protocol is found to be superior.

Additional treatments that have studies with positive results include medications, supplements, and acupuncture. There is not currently enough research looking at use of NSAIDs for more than just a short period of time to treat AIMSS. One study showed improvement in pain scores with use of duloxetine 60 mg daily [16]. Another study showed moderate improvement with glucosamine 1500 mg/day and chondroitin sulfate 1200 mg/day supplementation [17]. Finally, there have been several studies looking at the use of acupuncture for patients with diffuse AIMSS symptoms. Acupuncture is considered a safe and effective treatment. If symptoms are refractory, patients can discuss possibility of switching their aromatase inhibitor to another with their oncologist. Classically, the AIMSS symptoms should decrease/ resolve with cessation of the AI. For this reason, sometimes a drug holiday is recommended to confirm the cause of the symptoms prior to considering switching to a different medication.

Lymphedema is a frequently dreaded complication of cancer and cancer treatments; however, under the care of a knowledgeable clinician it can managed effectively in the vast majority of cases, and in some instances even prevented entirely. The disease is characterized by abnormal accumulation of lymphatic fluid, a protein-rich fluid normally carried by the lymphatic system, ultimately draining into lymphatic ducts or the venous system. Lymphedema is a result of a mechanical failure of this drainage system, resulting in impaired fluid transport. This fluid accumulates in the interstitium of the dermis and subcutaneous tissue. Fluid is effectively trapped in the tissues, meaning that lymphedema can be segmental in nature, not necessarily always a dependent edema, and does not respond as well to limb elevation as does cardiogenic edema, for example [18].

There are several major risk factors for lymphedema in cancer patients. One is the removal of lymph nodes (lymphadenectomy) that occurs in a lymph node dissection, as seen in breast cancer or melanoma, for example. Another is radiation to the axillary or pelvic nodes. Other risk factors include certain chemotherapies, obesity, and preexisting vascular issues [19, 20].

It is important for the clinician to understand the timing and incidence of lymphedema in this population as it can help guide clinical suspicion and aid in educating patients about their risk. Generally speaking, after sentinel lymph node biopsy (SLNB) the lifetime risk of developing lymphedema is less than 5%; radiation after SLNB doubles the risk to approximately 10%. Following axillary lymph node dissection (ALND) the risk increases to 20–30% and adding radiation gives a lifetime risk of 30–50%. Though these figures represent a lifetime risk, it is important to note that most patients who develop lymphedema (80%) will develop it within the first 2 years of their surgery [21]. Keeping these risk factors in mind can help guide a differential diagnosis of patient's localized edema.

Lymphedema is a treatable condition, but if left untreated has many significant sequalae including: discomfort and disfigurement, impaired use of the limb, permanent skin changes, and a predisposition to cellulitis. Monitoring of a lymphedema patient involves essentially monitoring for increases in swelling of the at-risk limb. This can be done with perometry, bioimpedance spectroscopy, or just circumferential measurements using a tape measure. Obtaining a baseline measurement prior to a lymph node dissection or other operation is recommended. Then periodic measurements can be done following surgery, which is particularly important during the highest risk periods. If the cause of the edema is unclear or the need exists to quantify the impaired lymphatic flow, lymphoscintigraphy is the gold standard imaging study.

If subclinical lymphedema is detected on bioimpedance spectroscopy or measurable edema develops with an increase in volume less than 8%, prophylactic donning of a lymphedema compression garment during the day has been shown to reverse the swelling. If the swelling is greater than 8% or is refractory to compression, the patient should be referred to a certified lymphedema therapist for complete decongestive therapy (CDT) [22]. CDT is a comprehensive approach and must include manual lymphatic drainage, multi-layer bandaging, and home exercise teaching. It must also include education regarding self-management, precautions, and skin care. Following CDT, patients typically are measured for lymphedema garments that must be worn daily to contain the limb and prevent fluid accumulation. Some patients also may benefit from home intermittent pneumatic compression pumps. While historically patients were instructed that exercise may precipitate lymphedema, this has been debunked and, in fact, the opposite is true. Exercising the affected limb is now routinely recommended [23, 24]. Compression is the standard of care for the treatment of lymphedema. However, should it be refractory, other emerging treatments can be explored. These include stellate ganglion blocks and lymphatic microsurgeries such as lymphovenous anastomosis or vascularized lymph node transfer.

Medical professionals are all familiar with fatigue. However, cancer-related fatigue (CRF) is a distinct pathological diagnosis. It is usually much more intense and differs from general fatigue in many ways. It is defined as a subjective sense of tiredness or exhaustion that is pervasive and interferes with daily activities. Importantly, it is characteristically not proportional to exertion and is not relieved by rest [25]. It may persist for months or years after successful treatment completion. It's believed to be the most frequent complaint in cancer patients, with an estimated prevalence of 60–90% [26]. Due to this extremely high prevalence, it is prudent for oncology providers to screen patients initially, throughout their cancer treatments, and on all follow-up visits.

While the etiology of CRF is poorly understood, it is almost certainly multifactorial in nature. Proinflammatory cytokines, impaired neuroendocrine regulation, and sleep-wake disturbances are some examples of proposed mechanisms, likely interacting in a feedback loop [27]. Regardless of cause, it is the role of the cancer rehabilitation practitioner to rule out other potentially contributing comorbidities. These include screening a patient for anemia, thyroid hypofunction, cardiac insufficiency, infections, and mood disorders. Fatigue as a side effect of medications (e.g., beta blockers, gabapentin) should be evaluated. It is prudent to attend to these as CRF is difficult to treat and these conditions are frequently reversible and can be more easily addressed.

The treatment with the highest level of scientific rigor is aerobic exercise. While many clinicians may feel it is hopeless to recommend exercise to a severely fatigued patient, studies have shown that patient compliance is good, particularly with supervised exercise sessions and with home-based walking programs [28]. The type, frequency, and intensity of recommended exercise varies in the literature, but most evidence points to moderate-intensity aerobic exercise with some evidence for resistance training [29]. Other nonpharmacological interventions include patient/family education, cognitive-behavioral therapy and energy conservation strategies as taught by physical or occupational therapists. Pharmacological interventions, used for refractory cases, include modafinil and methylphenidate [30, 31]. There is preliminary data that anti-proinflammatory cytokine therapies may be effective as well, representing an exciting new therapeutic option for this pervasive and debilitating complication of cancer and cancer treatment [32].

Clinical Case

A 63 year-old female is referred to you by a breast surgeon for right breast pain, right arm swelling, and diffuse joint pains. She has a history of locally advanced/inflammatory right-sided HER2 positive, ER negative, PR weakly-positive breast cancer currently with no evidence of disease. She is status post neoadjuvant chemotherapy with FEC/TPH(Fluorouracil, Epirubicin, and Cyclophosphamide followed by Docetaxel, Pertuzumab, and Trastuzumab/

Herceptin) followed by mastectomy and axillary lymph node dissection (2/35 lymph nodes involved), which showed residual disease within the breast and axilla. She has completed postmastectomy radiotherapy and maintenance Herceptin. A few months later she underwent revision of bilateral breasts and abdominal donor site, fat injection to bilateral breasts, left mastopexy, and right nipple reconstruction. She is currently on letrozole/Femara for chemoprevention.

Regarding right breast pain, she complains of maximal pain in the tail of the breast at the chest wall near the axilla. She describes the area of the surgical scar as "being hard like a rock," with "soreness" in the breast and axilla. The pain is worst when she goes to move or turn at which point she feels a "jabbing or stabbing" pain. She notes that she is unable to sleep on her right side. She also reports tingling and burning in the axilla and proximal posterior arm. She has not tried any medications or injections for this pain.

Regarding right arm swelling, she noted this about 8 months after her mastectomy and axillary lymph node dissection when she realized her rings started getting tight. She also notes that she has trouble reaching overhead with the affected arm.

Regarding joint pains, she has a history of joint pains in the past, however, these were amplified after starting letrozole, which she has taken for about the past 4 years. Maximum pain is in the knees and hands. In addition to pain she feels stiffness. In the past, she has tried meloxicam with some success.

Example treatment plan:

Right breast pain is likely musculoskeletal as well as neuropathic in nature. Physical therapy prescription is given for scar mobilization that will help break up the painful tissue in the breast and axilla. The neuropathic tingling and burning in the axilla and posterior arm is in the distribution of the intercostobrachial nerve, termed intercostobrachial neuralgia, for which a nerve block using ultrasound guidance is performed at the next visit.

Right arm swelling is a result of lymphedema. The timeframe of development in the first 6 months to 1 year postoperatively fits with this diagnosis. Prescription is given for complete decongestive therapy, to include bandaging, manual lymphatic drainage, exercise, and eventual garment fitting. The heaviness of the arm has resulted in disuse and she is developing adhesive capsulitis. This is addressed with injections and prescription for occupational therapy.

Joint pains are a result of her letrozole, resulting in aromatase-inhibitor-induced musculoskeletal symptoms (AIMSS). She likely had some degree of preexisting osteoarthritis in the affected joints, which is now exacerbated by the aromatase inhibitor. After examination, you prescribe a combination of NSAIDs, splinting, hand therapy, and corticosteroid injections. Once pain is better under control, she is given a home exercise program of moderate-intensity exercise.

Multiple Choice Questions

1. First-line treatment for cancer-related fatigue is:

    A. Cognitive-behavioral therapy
    B. Methylphenidate
    C. Modafinil
    D. Aerobic exercise
    E. Energy conservation strategies

2. Which of the following aspects of cancer treatments can increase the risk of developing lymphedema?

    A. Chemotherapy
    B. Radiation
    C. Weight gain from steroids
    D. Lymphadenectomy surgery
    E. All of the above

3. What is the most common site/location of involvement in AIMSS?

    A. Knees
    B. Ankles

C. Shoulders
D. Hands/wrists
E. Elbows

4. What are some diagnoses that can be associated with post-mastectomy pain syndrome?

A. Incisional pain
B. Rotator cuff syndrome
C. Axillary Web Syndrome
D. Intercostobrachial neuralgia
E. All of the above

Answers

1. D

While many in the medical community feel it is futile to recommend aerobic exercise to a severely fatigued patient, studies have shown that patient compliance is good, particularly with supervised exercise sessions and especially with home-based walking programs. Most evidence points to moderate-intensity aerobic exercise with some evidence for resistance training.

2. E

Certain chemotherapies, lymph node irradiation, obesity, and axillary or inguinal lymphadenectomy as part of cancer surgeries all have been proven to increase one's risk of developing lymphedema.

3. D

While symptoms of AIMSS can affect many different locations in the body, the most commonly reported area of involvement is the hands and wrists. The next most common location is the knees.

4. E

All of these syndromes/diagnoses can be the underlying cause of a patient's chest wall pain following breast surgery.

References

1. Annual Report to the Nation 2018, Part 1: National Cancer Statistics. CDC. Seer.cancer.gov
2. Ung O, Tan M, Chua B, Barraclough B. Complete axillary dissection: a technique that still has relevance in contemporary management of breast cancer. ANZ J Surg. 2006;76:518.
3. Ribnikar D, Sousa B, Cufer T, Cardoso F. Extended adjuvant endocrine therapy – a standard for all or some? Breast. 2017;32:112–8.
4. Anderson WF, Chatterjee N, Ershler WB, Brawley OW. Estrogen receptor breast cancer phenotypes in the Surveillance, Epidemiology, and End Results database. Breast Cancer Res Treat. 2002;76:27–36. https://doi.org/10.1023/A:1020299707510.
5. Lee YT. Breast carcinoma: pattern of metastasis at autopsy. J Surg Oncol. 1983;23(3):175–80.
6. Macdonald L, Bruce J, Scott NW, et al. Long-term follow up of breast cancer survivors with post-mastectomy pain syndrome. Br J Cancer. 2005;92(2):225–30.
7. Cheville A, et al. Adjunctive rehabilitation approaches to oncology. Phys Med Rehabil Clin N Am. 2017;28:153–69.
8. Belfer I, et al. Persistent postmastectomy pain in breast cancer survivors: analysis of clinical, demographic, and psychosocial factors. J Pain. 2013;14(10):1185–95.
9. Fourie WJ, Robb KA. Physiotherapy management of axillary web syndrome following breast cancer treatment: discussing the use of soft tissue techniques. Physiotherapy. 2009;95(4):314–20.
10. Shamley D, et al. Three-dimensional scapulothoracic motion following treatment for breast cancer. Breast Cancer Res Treat. 2009;118(2):315–22.
11. Lombard JM, Zdenkowski N, Wells K, Beckmore C, Reaby L, Forbes JF, Chirgwin J. Aromatase inhibitor induced musculoskeletal syndrome: a significant problem with limited treatment options. Support Care Cancer. 2016;24(5):2139–46.
12. Crew Katherine D, et al. Prevalence of joint symptoms in postmenopausal women taking aromatase inhibitors for early-stage breast cancer. J Clin Oncol. 2007;25(25):3877–83.
13. Castel LD, Hartmann KE, Mayer IA, Saville BR, Alvarez J, Boomershine CS, Abramson VG, Chakravarthy AB, Friedman DL, Cella DF. Time course of arthralgia among women initiating aromatase inhibitor therapy and a postmenopausal comparison group in a prospective cohort. Cancer. 2013;119(13):2375–82.

14. Stubblefield M, O'Dell M. Cancer rehabilitation: principles and practice. New York: Demos Medical; 2009.
15. Irwin ML, et al. Randomized exercise trial of aromatase inhibitor–induced arthralgia in breast cancer survivors. J Clin Oncol. 2015;33(10):1104–11.
16. Henry NL, Banerjee M, Wicha M, Van Poznak C, Smerage JB, Schott AF, Griggs JJ, Hayes DF. Pilot study of duloxetine for treatment of aromatase inhibitor-associated musculoskeletal symptoms. Cancer. 2011;117(24):5469–75.
17. Greenlee H, Crew KD, Shao T, Kranwinkel G, Kalinsky K, Maurer M, et al. Phase II study of glucosamine with chondroitin on aromatase inhibitor-associated joint symptoms in women with breast cancer. Support Care Cancer. 2013;21(4): 1077–87.
18. Rockson SG. Lymphedema. Am J Med. 2001;110(4):288–95.
19. Disipio T, Rye S, Newman B, Hayes S. Incidence of unilateral arm lymphoedema after breast cancer: a systematic review and meta-analysis. Lancet Oncol. 2013;14(6):500–15.
20. Shah C, Arthur D, Riutta J, Whitworth P, Vicini FA. Breast-cancer related lymphedema: a review of procedure-specific incidence rates, clinical assessment AIDS, treatment paradigms, and risk reduction. Breast J. 2012;18(4):357–61.
21. Norman SA, Localio AR, Potashnik SL, et al. Lymphedema in breast cancer survivors: incidence, degree, time course, treatment, and symptoms. J Clin Oncol. 2009;27(3):390–7.
22. Stout Gergich NL, Pfalzer LA, McGarvey C, Springer B, Gerber LH, Soballe P. Preoperative assessment enables the early diagnosis and successful treatment of lymphedema. Cancer. 2008;112(12):2809–19.
23. D'Egidio V, Sestili C, Mancino M, et al. Counseling interventions delivered in women with breast cancer to improve health-related quality of life: a systematic review. Qual Life Res. 2017;26(10):2573–92.
24. Rogan S, Taeymans J, Luginbuehl H, Aebi M, Mahnig S, Gebruers N. Therapy modalities to reduce lymphoedema in female breast cancer patients: a systematic review and meta-analysis. Breast Cancer Res Treat. 2016;159(1):1–14.
25. Berger AM, Gerber LH, Mayer DK. Cancer-related fatigue: implications for breast cancer survivors. Cancer. 2012;118(8 Suppl):2261–9.
26. Wagner LI, Cella D. Fatigue and cancer: causes, prevalence and treatment approaches. Br J Cancer. 2004;91(5):822–8.

27. Miller AH, Ancoli-Israel S, Bower JE, Capuron L, Irwin MR. Neuroendocrine-immune mechanisms of behavioral comorbidities in patients with cancer. J Clin Oncol. 2008;26(6):971–82.
28. Velhuis MJ, Agasi-Idenburg SC, Aufdemkampe G, Wittink HM. The effect of physical exercise on cancer-related fatigue during cancer treatment: a meta-analysis of randomised controlled trials. Clin Oncol (R Coll Radiol). 2010;22(3):208–21.
29. Stevinson C, Lawlor DA, Fox KR. Exercise interventions for cancer patients: systematic review of controlled trials. Cancer Causes Control. 2004;15(10):1035–56.
30. Minton O, Richardson A, Sharpe M, Hotopf M, Stone PC. Psychostimulants for the management of cancer-related fatigue: a systematic review and meta-analysis. J Pain Symptom Manag. 2011;41(4):761–7.
31. Jean-Pierre P, Morrow GR, Roscoe JA, et al. A phase 3 randomized, placebo-controlled, double-blind, clinical trial of the effect of modafinil on cancer-related fatigue among 631 patients receiving chemotherapy: a University of Rochester Cancer Center Community Clinical Oncology Program Research base study. Cancer. 2010;116(14):3513–20.
32. Monk JP, Phillips G, Waite R, et al. Assessment of tumor necrosis factor alpha blockade as an intervention to improve tolerability of dose-intensive chemotherapy in cancer patients. J Clin Oncol. 2006;24(12):1852–9.

Chapter 3
Cancer of the Digestive Organs: Importance of Mobility for Motility

An Ngo-Huang and George Francis

Introduction

Cancers of the digestive organs encompass a wide variety of malignancies throughout the course of the gastrointestinal (GI) tract. These include upper GI (oral, gastroesophageal, stromal) [1], lower GI (colorectal, anal) [2], hepatobiliary (gall bladder, liver, cholangiocarcinoma) [3], and pancreatic carcinomas [4]. Impairments in the head and neck region such as dysphagia, dysphonia, and radiation fibrosis of the neck are covered in separate chapters.

GI cancers are generally grouped into TNM staging (see Table 3.1) [5]. Colorectal cancers are most common, with approximately 150,000 people diagnosed yearly in the United States. As a result of excellent screening measures, they are often caught early and are cured through surgical resection [6]. Gastric and pancreatic cancer and cholangiocarcinoma, while less common, are often more aggressive. This results in poorer outcomes and decreased 5-year survival rates [7].

A. Ngo-Huang (✉)
Palliative, Rehabilitation, and Integrative Medicine, University of Texas MD Anderson Cancer Center, Houston, TX, USA
e-mail: ango2@mdanderson.org

G. Francis
Physical Medicine and Rehabilitation, Tom Baker Cancer Center, University of Calgary, Calgary, AB, Canada

© Springer Nature Switzerland AG 2020
J. Baima, A. Khanna (eds.), *Cancer Rehabilitation*,
https://doi.org/10.1007/978-3-030-44462-4_3

TABLE 3.1 TNM Staging of various GI malignancies according to the American Joint Committee on Cancer [5]

Pancreatic cancer	Esophageal cancer	Colon cancer
Primary tumor	*Primary tumor (T)*	*Tumor (T)*
Tx: primary tumor cannot be assessed	Tis: high-grade dysplasia	TX: primary tumor cannot be assessed
T0: no evidence of tumor	T1: invasion into lamina propria, muscularis	T0: no evidence of primary tumor
Tis: carcinoma in situ	mucosae, or submucosa	Tis: carcinoma in situ; intramucosal carcinoma (involvement of lamina propria with no extension through muscularis mucosae)
T1: tumor limited to pancreas, 2 cm or less in greatest dimension	T2: invasion into muscularis propria	T1: invades submucosa (through the muscularis mucosae but not into the muscularis propria)
T2: tumor limited to pancreas, more than 2 cm and less than 4 cm in greatest dimension	T3: invasion into adventitia	T2: invades muscularis propria
T3: tumor more than 4 cm in greatest dimension	T4a: invasion into resectable adjacent structures (e.g. pleura, pericardium, diaphragm)	T3: invades through muscularis propria into pericolorectal tissues
T4: tumor involves celiac axis, superior mesenteric artery, and/or common hepatic artery, regardless of size	T4b: invasion into unresectable adjacent structures (e.g., aorta, trachea, vertebral body)	T4: invades visceral peritoneum or invades or adheres to adjacent organ or structure
		T4a: invades through visceral peritoneum
		T4b: directly invades or adheres to adjacent organs or structures
Regional lymph nodes	*Nearby lymph nodes (N)*	*Regional lymph nodes (N)*
Nx: regional lymph nodes cannot be assessed	N0: no regional lymph node metastasis	NX: regional nodes cannot be assessed
N0: no regional lymph node metastasis	N1: 1 to 2 positive regional lymph nodes	N0: no regional node metastasis
N1: metastases in 1 to 3 regional lymph nodes	N2: 3 to 6 positive regional lymph nodes	N1: 1 to 3 regional nodes are positive (tumor in lymph nodes measuring 0.2 mm or more, or any number of tumor deposits are present and all identifiable lymph nodes are negative)
N2: metastases in 4 or more regional lymph nodes	N3: 7 or more positive regional lymph nodes	N1a: 1 regional node is positive
		N1b: 2 or 3 regional nodes are positive
		N1c: No regional nodes are positive, but there are tumor deposits in subserosa, mesentery, or nonperitonealized pericolic or perirectal/mesorectal tissues
		N2: 4 or more regional nodes are positive
		N2a: 4 to 6 regional nodes are positive
		N2b: 7 or more regional nodes are positive
Distant metastases	*Metastasis (M)*	*Distant metastases (M)*
M0: no distant metastases	M0: no distant metastasis	M0: no distant metastasis
M1: distant metastasis	M1: distant metastasis	M1: metastasis to 1 or more distant sites or organs, or peritoneal metastasis is identified
		M1a: metastasis to 1 site or organ without peritoneal metastasis
		M1b: metastases to 2 or more sites or organs without peritoneal metastasis
		M1c: metastasis to peritoneal surface alone or with other site or organ metastases

As with other cancer types, GI cancers may be treated with a combination of surgery, chemotherapy/immunotherapy, and radiation therapy. They present several rehabilitation challenges along the cancer continuum of care.

Diagnosis

At the time of diagnosis, GI cancers may have already caused bowel dysfunction, abdominal pain, generalized weakness, and cachexia [8]. Further cancer rehabilitation challenges for this population include: deconditioning, profound muscle loss due to cachexia, cancer-related fatigue, cancer pain, peripheral neuropathy, bowel and bladder dysfunction, gait abnormality, impairment in self-care, insomnia, anorexia, malnutrition, and concomitant mood disorders (adjustment disorders, anxiety, and depressed mood.) Thus, the involvement of a physiatrist early after cancer diagnosis is important to provide supportive care through symptom management, optimization of physical function, and monitoring of body composition changes during treatment.

Prior to surgical or chemotherapeutic treatment, optimization of performance status through prehabilitation is very important to reduce peri- and post-treatment complications, morbidity, and hospital length of stay [9]. Measures including presence of cachexia, sarcopenia, and/or malnutrition [10], hand grip strength [11], gait speed [12], and the six-minute walk test [13] have all been demonstrated to have predictive value in terms of postsurgical outcomes.

Prehabilitation has been shown to be feasible in several GI malignancies, including colon [14], pancreatic [15], and esophageal [16, 17] carcinomas. Prehabilitation may involve one (unimodal) or multiple elements (multimodal), including physical conditioning through exercise, nutrition optimization, or psychological interventions. The goals of physical prehabilitation are to optimize functional status, cardiovascular fitness, and muscle mass prior to intense cancer treatment and its anticipated side effects. Unfortunately, there is no standardized prehabilitation plan, as treatment protocols differ between various cancer types and centers.

Physical prehabilitation typically consists of a combination of aerobic and resistance exercises, with general recommendations for 150 minutes of moderate-intensity aerobic exercisely weekly and two sessions resistance exercises each week [18]. Personalization of an exercise program is important if patients have musculoskeletal or neuromuscular impairments that interfere with the ability to exercise. Implementation of these exercise prescriptions may vary: home-based exercise administered by a physiotherapist or exercise physiologist, skilled physiotherapy (PT) and occupational therapy (OT) if patient requires more guidance, supervised group exercises at a wellness center, or exercise with a certified exercise trainer. Nutritional support is a key component of prehabilitation as protein supplementation aids in muscle protein synthesis. Aim is for 1.2–2.0 g of protein/kilogram weight per day, depending on comorbidities [16, 19]. If available, consultation with a clinical dietitian is highly recommended soon after diagnosis of a GI cancer given the high risk of cachexia and malnutrition in this patient population.

Treatment

Treatment varies depending on tumor location and stage, and may include surgery, neoadjuvant or adjuvant chemoradiotherapy, immunotherapy, or a combination of any of the above. Surgical resection of GI cancer is often an extensive procedure, such as complete gastrectomy, pancreaticoduodenectomy, or abdominoperineal resection. A bowel ostomy may or may not be required. Patients receiving resection for an upper GI cancer may require enteral tube feeding. Following these invasive surgical procedures, deep venous thrombosis (DVT) risk is high, and prophylaxis is warranted [20]. Immediate postoperative mobility programs are highly encouraged – patients are advised to ambulate on the first postoperative day and have all initial meals out of bed. An abdominal binder may be helpful for transfers and during ambulation. Lifting precautions are generally restricted to 5–10 pounds for 6 weeks postoperatively for major abdominal surgeries. Home health services may be necessary initially for skilled nursing to monitor drains, to aid in tube feeding and/or ostomy management, and the patient may require PT and/or OT. Deconditioning and cachexia may occur (or worsen from preoperative states). Thus, ongoing physical rehabilitation through a walking program or other aerobic exercise and resistance exercise is important in maximizing function and preventing further deconditioning postoperatively [21].

Chemotherapeutic agents utilized in GI cancers include fluorouracil, leucovorin, taxanes, platinum agents, capecitabine, gemcitabine, and biologic therapies [22]. Common side effects of these chemotherapies are listed in Table 3.2. Radiation is often part of treatment and can further exacerbate cachexia due to nausea, vomiting, and anorexia [23]. Patients should be monitored regularly for low blood counts that may warrant exercise precautions due to risk of falls and hemorrhage [24, 25]. Restrictions on resistance exercises are recommended with platelet counts below 20,000 per microliter and walking is encouraged for this population with monitoring of symptoms [25]. For patients with significant anemia (hemoglobin ≤8 grams per deciliter), a symptom-based approach to exercise is advised with extra precaution with moderate- to high-intensity exercise [25]. (For more information on specific restrictions related to blood counts, see chapter on hematologic malignancies.)

Furthermore, monitoring of skin is important to prevent the development of ulcers due to peripheral neuropathy. Adequate fiber and fluid intake along with bowel medications will help manage diarrhea [26]. Radiation side effects including radiation dermatitis, muscle fibrosis, and myoneuropathy should be promptly evaluated and targeted with a range of motion exercises and manual therapy. Lastly, mobility through a daily walking program throughout the treatment and post-treatment period reduces the risk of DVT formation and pulmonary complications [27] while improving function, fatigue, and sleep quality [28].

TABLE 3.2 Common side effects of chemotherapies [39–45]

Chemotherapy drug	Function-impacting side effects
5-Fluorouracil	Acute cerebellar syndrome, anorexia, confusion, esophagitis, headache, insomnia, nausea and vomiting, pancytopenia, thromboembolism
Irinotecan	Abdominal pain, back pain, bleeding, bradycardia, constipation, diaphoresis, dizziness, drowsiness, edema, fever, insomnia, muscle cramps, orthostatic hypotension and syncope, vertigo
Oxaliplatin & Cisplatin	Abdominal pain, anorexia, anxiety, arthralgias, ataxia, back and bone pain, cranial nerve palsies, dizziness, dysarthria, dysphagia, fatigue, hearing loss, insomnia, myalgias, peripheral neuropathy, pulmonary fibrosis, seizures, thrombocytopenia, urinary incontinence, vertigo, weakness
Leucovorin	Agitation, dehydration, diarrhea, insomnia, nausea, seizures, syncope, vomiting
Docetaxel & Paclitaxel	Abdominal pain, anorexia, arthralgias, asthenia, back pain, bronchospasm, confusion, dizziness, dysesthesia, dyspnea, fatigue, hearing loss, myalgias, neurotoxicity, peripheral edema, peripheral neuropathy, seizures, syncope, thrombocytopenia, vomiting, weight change

Note that these are not comprehensive lists and focus on function-impacting adverse effects

Survivorship

Five-year survivorship rates vary from less than 10% for pancreatic ductal adenocarcinoma [29] up to 100% for rectal T1 carcinoid tumors [30]. Long-term rehabilitative and functional issues affecting GI cancer survivors include fecal incontinence [31], neuropathy induced by chemotherapy and vitamin B12 deficiency [32], cognitive changes, sexual dysfunction [33], bone pain, and neurologic weakness including foot drop. While musculoskeletal and neurologic metastases are less common in GI cancers, diligence in monitoring neuromuscular function will aid in early diagnosis and prompt intervention. For example, treatment of neuropathy can include thorough education, daily foot inspection, and topical and/or oral neuropathic agents [34].

Furthermore, since an ostomy may be required for bowel emptying, perioperative disruption of bowel function and the nonuse of pelvic and core musculature may result in decreased muscle bulk and coordination in sphincter control [35]. This may be detrimental in the case of an ostomy reversal in survivorship, as patients may have fecal incontinence. It may also result in difficulty with core stability, transfers, and chronic back pain secondary to poor posture [36]. Ongoing physical rehabilitation including core strengthening, pelvic floor exercises, pelvic floor rehabilitation and frequent ambulation manages these symptoms, while at the same time maximizing function, quality of life, and possibly survival [37, 38].

Clinical Case

A 68-year-old woman with history of esophagectomy and graft for bleeding varices at age 15 had an anemia workup that revealed adenocarcinoma of the colon interposition. She received neoadjuvant chemotherapy and underwent a right thoracotomy, esophagectomy, resection of the colon interposition, gastrectomy, lymphadenectomy, jejunostomy, feeding tube, and lysis of adhesions. She had a complicated postoperative course with respiratory failure, atrial fibrillation, severe malnutrition, poorly controlled pain (history of rheumatoid arthritis), and depression. She was admitted to acute inpatient rehabilitation to focus on household ambulation and ADL training, including management of her ostomy bags and tube feeds. Barriers to rehabilitation included: severe sarcopenia, malnutrition, poor wound healing, cancer-related fatigue, depression, psychosocial concerns (her husband was diagnosed with metastatic cancer), and body image concerns (esophagostomy prominent in her upper chest). She was discharged from inpatient rehabilitation to home at a supervision level for activities of daily living (ADLs) and gait distance of 500 feet.

Three months later, she returned to the PM&R clinic requesting to be "put back together." Her surgeons were concerned about her poor tolerance for surgery and recommended improvement in her functional, nutrition, and psychological status.

She was initiated on a multimodal prehabilitation program that included:

- Aerobic exercise: walking or recumbent bicycling 30 minutes per day
- Resistance exercises engaging major muscle groups twice a week
- Individualized clinical dietitian intervention
- Ongoing psychotherapy with a psychologist

Her depression was treated with cognitive behavioral therapy, which was integral to her individualized prehabilitation program. She was highly compliant with the exercise program: walked 1–2 miles per day, performing 40 sit-to-stands consecutively, and at the end of a six-week intervention, had improved functional scores, with some values better than age-related norms.

She underwent the second surgery: laparotomy, reversal of the esophageal discontinuity, hemimanubrectomy, jejunojejunostomy, and flaps for closure. During the postoperative PT evaluation, she was at modified independent level for bed mobility, transfers, and ambulated 400 feet without an assistive device. She had no major complications and was discharged to home 7 days postoperatively. She did not require home health or outpatient rehabilitation.

She continues to make progress with a home-based exercise program of daily walking, resistance exercises, and water aerobics. She remains engaged in her local community and on her farm.

TABLE 3.3 Summary of functional impairment and rehabilitation diagnoses at Diagnosis, Treatment and Survivorship

Timeline of Cancer	Functional impairment and rehabilitation diagnoses
Diagnosis	Anorexia and cachexia, sarcopenia, cancer-related fatigue, deconditioning, cancer-pain, bowel dysfunction, mood disorders.
Treatment	Postoperative deconditioning, cancer-related fatigue, cancer-pain, peripheral neuropathy, malnutrition, chemotherapy and radiation side effects, decreased mobility, impaired ADLs, mood disorders.
Survivorship	Muscle weakness, reduced muscle mass, cognitive dysfunction, mood disorders, peripheral neuropathy, chronic cancer-related pain and neuropathic pain, imbalance, and bowel, bladder, and sexual dysfunction.

Conclusion

GI cancers may vary widely with respect to location, progression, and treatment, but cause several impairments that affect the overall status of the patient. The implementation of rehabilitation includes prehabilitation at diagnosis, continued physical activity and optimized nutrition during treatment, appropriate referral for symptom management, and maintenance of strength and endurance in survivorship. Proper nutrition and core and pelvic floor strengthening are of particular importance in this population. Physiatry involvement in the management of these patients is important at each stage of treatment, as summarized in Table 3.3.

Multiple Choice Questions

1. Which of the following tumor types is not classified as a hepatobiliary carcinoma?

   A. Pancreatic
   B. Gallbladder

   C. Cholangiocarcinoma
   D. Liver

2. A colorectal tumor that has invaded completely through the muscularis propria and has affected one lymph node would be classified as:

   A. T2N1M0
   B. T3N0M1
   C. T3N1M0
   D. T4N1M0

3. Research supports evidence for prehabilitation for which of the following GI malignancies?

   A. Colorectal
   B. Gastroesophageal
   C. Pancreatic
   D. All of the above

4. Which of the following is not a common potential side effect of FOLFOX (fluorouracil, leucovorin, oxaliplatin) chemotherapy?

   A. Peeling of the palms/soles
   B. Peripheral neuropathy
   C. Xerostomia
   D. Fever

5. Which of the following statements is false?

   A. Chemotherapy-induced neuropathy requires multi-modal management including physical therapy, medications and preventive measures.
   B. Musculoskeletal metastases are common in colorectal cancer.
   C. Pelvic floor strengthening improves sphincter function and quality of life.
   D. Regular ambulation improves gastric motility.

Answers

1. A
2. C
3. D
4. C
5. B

References

1. Gore RM, Mehta UK, Berlin JW, Rao V, Newmark GM. Upper gastrointestinal tumours: diagnosis and staging. Cancer Imaging. 2006;6(1):213–7.
2. Gore RM. Lower gastrointestinal tract tumours: diagnosis and staging strategies. Cancer Imaging. 2005;5:S140–3.
3. National Comprehensive Cancer Network. Hepatobiliary cancers: clinical practice guidelines in oncology. J Nat Comp Cancer Network. 2009;7(4):350–91.
4. Mostafa ME, Erbarut-Seven I, Pehlivanoglu B, Adsay V. Pathologic classification of "pancreatic cancers" current concepts and challenges. Chin Clin Oncol. 2017;6(6):59.
5. American Joint Committee on Cancer. AJCC cancer staging manual. 8th ed. Cham: Springer; 2017.
6. American Cancer Society. Colorectal cancer facts & figures 2017–2019. Atlanta: American Cancer Society; 2017.
7. Surveillance, Epidemiology, and End Results (SEER) Program (www.seer.cancer.gov) Research Data (1973–2015), National Cancer Institute, DCCPS, Surveillance Research Program, released April 2018, based on the November 2017 submission.
8. Palesty JA, Dudrick SJ. What we have learned about cachexia in gastrointestinal cancer. Dig Dis. 2003;21(3):198–213.
9. Silver JK, Baima J. Cancer prehabilitation: an opportunity to decrease treatment-related morbidity, increase cancer treatment options, and improve physical and psychological health outcomes. Am J Phys Med Rehabil. 2013;2(8):715–27.
10. Fukuta A, Saito T, Murata S, Makiura D, Inoue J, Okumura M, Sakai Y, Ono R. Impact of preoperative cachexia on postoperative length of stay in elderly patients with gastrointestinal cancer. Nutrition. 2019;58:65–8.

11. Sato S, Nagai E, Taki Y, Watanabe M, Watanabe Y, Nakano K, Yamada H, Chiba T, Ishii Y, Ogiso H, Takagi M. Hand grip strength as a predictor of postoperative complications in esophageal cancer patients undergoing esophagectomy. Esophagus. 2018;15(1):10–8.
12. Chandoo A, Chi C-H, Ji W, Huang Y, Chen X-D, Zhang W-T, Wu R-S, Shen X. Gait speed predicts post-operative medical complications in elderly gastric patients following gastrectomy. ANZ J Surg. 2017;88:723–6.
13. Awdeh H, Kassak K, Sfeir P, Hatoum H, Bitar H, Husari A. The SF-36 and 6-minute walk test are significant predictors of complications after major surgery. World J Surg. 2015;39(6):1406–12.
14. Minnella EM, Carli F. Prehabilitation and functional recovery for colorectal cancer patients. Eur J Surg Oncol. 2018;44(7):919–26.
15. Parker NH, Ngo-Huang A, Lee RE, O'Connor DP, Basen-Engquist KM, Petzel MQB, Wang X, Xiao L, Fogelman DR, Schadler KL, Simpson RJ, Fleming JB, Lee JE, Varadhachary GR, Sahai SK, Katz MHG. Physical activity and exercise during preoperative pancreatic cancer treatment. Support Care Cancer. 2018;27:4493–6.
16. Minnella EM, Awasthi R, Loiselle SE, Agnihotram RV, Ferri LE, Carli F. Effect of exercise and nutrition prehabilitation on functional capacity in esophagogastric cancer surgery. JAMA Surg. 2018;153(12):1081–9.
17. Dewberry LC, Wingrove LJ, Marsh MD, Glode AE, Schefter TE, Leong S, Purcell WT, McCarter MD. Pilot prehabilitation program for patients with esophageal cancer during neoadjuvant therapy and surgery. J Surg Res. 2019;235:66–72.
18. American Cancer Society. American Cancer Society guidelines on nutrition and physical activity for cancer survivors, 2012.
19. Carli F, Gillis C, Scheede-Bergdahl C. Promoting a culture of prehabilitation for the surgical cancer patient. Acta Oncol. 2017;56(2):128–33.
20. Toledano TH, Kondal D, Kahn SR, Tagalakis V. The occurrence of venous thromboembolism in cancers patients following major surgery. Thromb Res. 2013;131(1):e1–5.
21. van der Leeden M, Huijsmans R, Gelejin E, de Lange-de Klerk ES, Dekker J, Bonjer HJ, van der Peet DL. Early enforced mobilisation following surgery for gastrointestinal cancer: feasibility and outcomes. Physiotherapy. 2016;102(1):103–10.
22. Neuzillet C, Rousseau B, Kocher H, Bourget P, Tournigand C. Unravelling the pharmacologic opportunities and future

directions for targeted therapies in gastro-intestinal cancers Part 1: GI carcinomas. Pharmacol Ther. 2017;174:145–72.
23. Grabenbauer GG, Holger G. Management of radiation and che-motherapy related acute toxicity in gastrointestinal cancer. Best Pract Res Clin Gastroenterol. 2016;30(4):655–64.
24. Ghosn M, Farhat F, Kattan J, Younges F, Moukadem W, Nasr F, Chahine G. FOLFOX-6 combination as the first-line treatment of locally advanced and/or metastatic pancreatic cancer. Am J Clin Oncol. 2007;30(1):15–20.
25. Maltser S, Cristian A, Silver JK, Morris GS, Stout NL. A focused review of safety considerations in cancer rehabilitation. PM R. 2017;9(9S2):S415–28.
26. Andreyev J, Ross P, Donnellan C, Lennan E, Leonard P, Waters C, Wedlake L, Bridgewater J, Glynne-Jones R, Allum W, Chau I, Wilson R, Ferry D. Guidance on the management of diarrhoea during cancer chemotherapy. Lancet Oncol. 2014;15(10):e447–60.
27. Santos DA, Alseidi A, Shannon VR, Messick C, Song G, Ledet CR, Lee H, Ngo-Huang A, Francis G, Asher A. Management of surgical challenges in actively treated cancer patients. Curr Probl Surg. 2017;54(12):612–54.
28. Cheville AL, Kollasch J, Vandenberg J, Shen T, Grothey A, Gamble G, Basford JR. A home-based exercise program to improve function, fatigue, and sleep quality in patients with Stage IV lung and colorectal cancer: a randomized controlled trial. Pain Symptom Manage. 2013;45:811–21.
29. Balachandran VP, Beatty GL, Dougan SK. Broadening the impact of immunotherapy to pancreatic cancer: chal-lenges and opportunities. Gastroenterology. 2019; S0016-5085(19)30054–X. E-pub.
30. Ngamruengphong S, Kamal A, Akshintala V, Hajiyeva G, Hanada Y, Chen YI, Sanaei O, Fluxa D, Haito Chavez Y, Kumbhari V, Singh V, O'Broin-Lennon AM, Canto MI, Khashab MA. Prevalence of metastasis and survival of 788 patients with T1 rectal carcinoid tumors. Gastrointest Endosc. 2018;S0016-5107(1):33272–3. Epub.
31. Lin KY, Denehy L, Frawley HC, Wilson L, Granger CL. Pelvic floor symptoms, physical, and psychological outcomes of patients following surgery for colorectal cancer. Physiother Theory Pract. 2018;34(6):442–52.
32. Mols F, Beijers AJ, Vreugdenhil G, Verhulst A, Schep G, Husson O. Chemotherapy-induced peripheral neuropathy, physical activity and health-related quality of life among colorectal

cancer survivors from the PROFILES registry. J Cancer Surviv. 2015;9(3):512–22.

33. Frick MA, Vachani CC, Hampshire MK, Bach C, Arnold-Kozeniowski K, Metz JM, Hill-Kayser CE. Survivorship after lower gastrointestinal cancer: patient-reported outcomes and planning for care. Cancer. 2017;123(1):1860–8.

34. Jones MR, Urits I, Wolf J, Corrigan D, Colburn L, Peterson E, Williamson A, Viswanath O. Drug-induced peripheral neuropathy, a narrative review. Curr Clin Pharmacol. 2020;15(1):38–48.

35. Nishigori H, Ishii M, Kokado Y, Fujimoto K, Higashiyama H. Effectiveness of pelvic floor rehabilitation for bowel dysfunction after intersphincteric resection for lower rectal cancer. World J Surg. 2018;42(10):3415–21.

36. Herrle F, Sandra-Petrescu F, Weiss C, Post S, Runkel N, Kienle P. Quality of life and timing of stoma closure in patients with rectal cancer undergoing low anterior resection with diverting stoma: a Multicenter Longitudinal Observational Study. Dis Colon Rectum. 2016;59(4):281–90.

37. Zimmer P, Trebing S, Timmers-Trebing U, Schenk A, Paust R, Bloch W, Rudolph R, Streckmann F, Baumann FT. Eight-week, multimodal exercise counteracts a progress of chemotherapy-induced peripheral neuropathy and improves balance and strength in metastasized colorectal cancer patients: a randomized controlled trial. Support Care Cancer. 2018;6(2):615–24.

38. Van Blarigan EL, Fuchs CS, Niedzwiecki D, et al. Association of survival with adherence to the American Cancer Society nutrition and physical activity guidelines for cancer survivors after colon cancer diagnosis: the CALGB 89803/alliance trial. JAMA Oncol. 2018;4(6):783–90.

39. Fluorouracil, 5-FU. Drug monographs. ClinicalKey. Elsevier, Inc., Atlanta. Available at: https://www.clinicalkey.com. Accessed 14 Feb 2019.

40. Irinotecan. Drug monographs. ClinicalKey. Elsevier, Inc., Atlanta. Available at: https://www.clinicalkey.com. Accessed 14 Feb 2019.

41. Oxaliplatin. Drug monographs. ClinicalKey. Elsevier, Inc., Atlanta. Available at: https://www.clinicalkey.com. Accessed 14 Feb 2019.

42. Cisplatin. Drug monographs. ClinicalKey. Elsevier, Inc., Atlanta. Available at: https://www.clinicalkey.com. Accessed 14 Feb 2019.

43. Leucovorin. Drug monographs. ClinicalKey. Elsevier, Inc., Atlanta. Available at: https://www.clinicalkey.com. Accessed 14 Feb 2019.
44. Docetaxel. Drug monographs. ClinicalKey. Elsevier, Inc., Atlanta. Available at: https://www.clinicalkey.com. Accessed 14 Feb 2019.
45. Paclitaxel. Drug monographs. ClinicalKey. Elsevier, Inc. Atlanta. Available at: https://www.clinicalkey.com. Accessed 14 Feb 2019.

Chapter 4
Cancer of the Brain, Eye, and Other Parts of the Central Nervous System

Mary Vargo

Primary central nervous system (CNS) malignancies comprise just 1.4% of all cancers [1], and benign brain tumors have an incidence more than double that of malignant primary brain tumors (69.1% versus 30.9%) [2]. Brain and spinal metastatic disease greatly outnumber primary brain or spinal cord tumors [3]. Tumor types which commonly metastasize to brain include lung, breast, kidney, colorectal, and melanoma, affecting an estimated 20% of cancer patients [4]. In general, 2% of all nonhematologic cancer patients exhibit brain metastasis at the time of diagnosis [3]. Spine metastasis etiologies include breast, prostate, renal, and lung [5], affecting 5–10% of patients with advanced cancer [6].

Brain Tumor

The most common types of brain tumors are meningioma (36.8%), glioblastoma multiforme (GBM) (14.7%), pitu-

M. Vargo (✉)
Metro Health Medical Center, Department of Physical Medicine and Rehabilitation, Case Western Reserve University, Cleveland, OH, USA
e-mail: mvargo@metrohealth.org

© Springer Nature Switzerland AG 2020
J. Baima, A. Khanna (eds.), *Cancer Rehabilitation*,
https://doi.org/10.1007/978-3-030-44462-4_4

45

itary tumors (16.4%), and nerve sheath tumors (8.5%) [2]. The most common CNS tumor locations are meninges (37.2%), followed by pituitary and craniopharyngeal duct (17.5%), frontal lobe (8.2%), cranial nerves (7%), temporal lobe (6%), parietal lobe (3.5%), spinal cord (3.1%), cerebellum (2.2%), brainstem (1.5%), and occipital lobe (1%) [2].

While most brain tumors occur in the adult population, with median age of 60 [2], brain tumors are also the most common neoplasm occurring in childhood (age 0–14 years) [2]. Pediatric tumors are more likely to affect the posterior fossa and have different histologies. In the 0–14 age group, most common types include pilocytic astrocytoma (17.9%), malignant glioma (13.9%), and embryonal tumors (13.3%, with medulloblastoma comprising 62.4% of those). Prognosis varies with histology and in general is poorer with advancing age. Five-year survival of childhood malignant brain tumors is about 70%, compared to about 35% for adult brain tumors. Table 4.1 provides further details regarding survival rates by brain tumor type.

The incidence of disabling complications is reported at about 80% [7], with the most common impairments among rehabilitation inpatients being cognitive deficits (80%), weakness (78%), and visual-perceptual deficits (53%) [8]. Table 4.2 summarizes common patterns of weakness due to cancer-related central or peripheral nervous system abnormalities. Long-term survivors of childhood cancers have higher obesity rates than peers, and may experience effects on growth and other aspects of endocrine function [9]. In general, brain tumors have among the highest rates of impact on work [10] and school [11] performance.

Surgery is the mainstay of treatment. Major complications have an incidence of 13–16%, morbidity of 25–32%, and mortality of 1.7%. Risk factors include age >60, Karnofsky Performance Scale score less than or equal to 50, intraoperative bleeding, and posterior fossa location [12, 13]. Radiation therapy is often employed, usually external beam radiation, localized to the tumor via 3D mapping. Whole brain radiation may be used for metastatic tumors. Specialized radiation therapy techniques include stereotactic radiation with gamma

TABLE 4.1 Survival rates (%) by brain tumor type

Type of tumor	1 year	5 years	10 years
Meningioma (nonmalignant)	92.6	86.7	81.5
Meningioma (malignant)	82.1	63.8	56.1
Glioblastoma	40.2	5.6	2.8
Anaplastic astrocytoma	55	19.8	13.1
Diffuse astrocytoma	74.9	50.4	39.3
Pilocytic astrocytoma	97.9	94.1	92.2
Oligodendroglioma	94.7	81.6	66.3
Anaplastic oligodendroglioma	84.4	57.6	44.1
Ependymoma (nonmalignant)	97.9	97.4	96.6
Ependymoma (malignant)	94.4	84.8	79.5
Embryonal tumors	81.9	62.1	55.1
Medulloblastoma	89.3	73.2	64.9
PNET	75.3	46.4	40.8
Lymphoma	53.6	34.5	26.6
Nerve sheath tumors	99.4	99.3	99.3
Germ cell tumors	95	94.6	92.0
Pituitary tumors	98	96.6	94.6
Craniopharyngioma	92.8	83.5	77.7
Hemangioma	96.3	93.4	90.2

Adapted from Ostrum [2]

knife, brachytherapy (implanted radiation sources), and proton beam therapy [14]. Delayed radiation effects such as immediate and delayed radiation encephalopathy or radiation necrosis may complicate the clinical picture (Table 4.3), and must also be distinguished from progressive disease [15, 16].

For GBM, the most common chemotherapy is temozolamide, with side effects including fatigue, headache, and constipation. Patients on temozolamide may exhibit "pseudoprogression" on

TABLE 4.2 Weakness due to cancer-related central or peripheral nervous system abnormalities

Type of lesion	Usual presentation	Associated features
Brain tumor	Unilateral	Contralateral for cerebral involvement, may be ipsilateral for brainstem tumors
Brain radiation necrosis	Unilateral	Delayed presentation, up to a year or more
Meningeal carcinomatosis	Bilateral	Metastatic from hematologic, lung, breast, melanoma, gastric; poor prognosis
Spinal cord (neoplasm; post-radiation)	Bilateral	Back pain is most often the presenting clinical feature; paraplegia much more common than tetraplegia; thoracic level most common; motor change often precedes sensory
Nerve root invasion	Unilateral	Need to distinguish from plexopathy, radiation effect
Plexopathy (neoplasm; post-radiation)	Unilateral	Tumor invasion typically more painful than radiation plexopathy. Myokymia often seen on electromyography post-radiation.
Myopathy (carcinomatous; corticosteroid or other endocrine)	Bilateral	Exercise is mainstay in the prevention and treatment of corticosteroid myopathy [10].
Neuromuscular junction disorder	Bilateral	Rare. Presynaptic disorder may be seen in small cell lung cancer. Myasthenia gravis (postsynaptic disorder) in association with thymoma.
Peripheral polyneuropathy	Bilateral	Chemotherapy-associated is more common than primary neoplastic/paraneoplastic
Deconditioning	Bilateral	Rule out other neuromuscular pathology

imaging, with or without clinical deterioration [15]. Other agents include angiogenesis inhibitors such as bevacizumab. Novel therapies include NovoTTF-100A, an electrical field therapy applied via disposable transducers to the scalp for inhibiting cell growth, and immunotherapies such as vaccine-based approaches, as well as oncolytic virotherapy [14].

Steroids are almost universally used in the treatment of brain tumors, and nearly all brain tumor patients will receive glucocorticoids at some point in their treatment. Generally, they are administered to counteract treatment-related vaso-genic edema. For example, they are frequently used during radiation treatment. The most common is dexamethasone

TABLE 4.3 Cognition and cancer

Type of lesion	Usual presentation	Other
Brain tumor	Linked to tumor size and location [46]; 90% of patients with frontal or temporal lobe tumors pretreatment display impairments in at least one area of cognition [55]	Possible impact of epilepsy and/or epilepsy medications [16]. Often milder, more diffuse than in stroke patients, but still side specific [16]. Endocrine dysfunction.
Radiation encephalopathy	Acute (1–3 months) reversible clinical worsening Early delayed (3–12 months) "somnolence syndrome", most common and severe if age <3 years Syndrome of pseudoprogression (radiographic ± clinical) in association with temozolamide treatment Late delayed (>1 year), nonspecific clinical worsening [11]	Acute encephalopathy is related to swelling and treated with corticosteroids. Early delayed related to demyelination from injury to oligodentrocytes, can also be treated with corticosteroids. Both of these are less common with modern protocols. Late-delayed is related to vasculopathy, also treated with corticosteroids but may not be responsive, sometimes resection. Distinguish from recurrence, with advanced imaging such as PET [11].

(continued)

TABLE 4.3 (continued)

Type of lesion	Usual presentation	Other
Long-term cognitive change after whole brain radiation(diffuse cerebral injury)	Radiation-induced cognitive impairment reported in 50–90% of tumor survivors; deficits including processing speed, attention, learning, memory, and executive functions [46]. Cognitive changes most apparent in young children and elderly [11, 16]. Among children, lower IQ compared to age peers. In children with history of posterior fossa tumor, effects on academic ability, social skills, and attention, but not psychological distress or behavior problems [30]. In severe cases in adults, progressive dementia and altered gait [11]	Diffuse atrophy, ventriculomegaly, white matter signal abnormalities on imaging [11]. "Mineralizing microangiopathy" also occurs in up to one-third of children, consisting of calcifications in the basal ganglia, dentate nuclei, and cerebral gray-white matter junction [11]. RT is the most important risk factor for impaired intellectual outcome in childhood brain tumor [42].
Cancer-treatment-associated cognitive change	Effects on executive function, learning and memory, attention, and processing speed [8]	Probably multifactorial – neurotoxicity of treatments (especially chemotherapy); effects including diffuse white matter changes on neuroimaging, proinflammatory cytokine effects, possible effect of underlying tumor. Concurrent fatigue, anxiety, insomnia may heighten cognitive symptoms. Diminished prefrontal cortex blood flow in neuroimaging studies of breast cancer survivors who received chemotherapy [4].

due to its low mineralocorticoid activity, although methyl-prednisolone and prednisone are also used. The steroids are tapered down until the minimum effective dose is found. This is the dose at which the patient's symptom burden and deleterious effects of prolonged steroid use are minimized, while the functional ability of the patient is maximized. Some of these adverse effects include steroid-induced myopathy, which is embodied by proximal weakness, particularly in the hip girdle. Steroids also have a wasting effect on bone because of impaired calcium absorption, which can result in fractures or avascular necrosis of the hip. Calcium and vitamin D supplementation can be beneficial [16, 17].

Inpatient rehabilitation studies of brain tumor patients have consistently reported comparable functional outcomes and discharge to community rates as other brain rehabilitation populations, such as brain injury and stroke patients [18] (Table 4.4). However, interrupted stay is more common in the brain tumor patient (17–35% rates reported). In most series, there is no significant difference in rehabilitation outcomes between those with benign and malignant disease, or even those with metastatic disease, who do well in the near term [19].

Limited outpatient interdisciplinary outcome data for malignant brain tumor patients suggests favorable functional outcomes [20] and cost-effectiveness [21]. Cognitive rehabili-

TABLE 4.4 Inpatient rehabilitation compared to noncancer patients with similar impairment type

	Brain tumor	Spinal cord neoplasm
FIM gain	Similar or slightly less	Less
FIM efficiency	Similar	Similar
Rehabilitation length of stay	Similar or shorter	Shorter
Discharge to community	Similar	Similar
Interrupted stay	Higher	Higher

tation has been studied in various populations, including those with childhood tumors, and adult glioma patients [19], with recommendation for cognitive therapy as a practice guideline for children and adolescents treated for brain tumor [22]. Studies of methylphenidate, memantine, or done-pezil have shown benefits in cognitive performance, to a varying extent [19].

There is evidence that physical activity is of benefit. Among a cohort of 243 recurrent malignant glioma patients, self-reported exercise level of >9 MET-h/week was associated with survival of nearly 22 months, versus 13 months among the less active [23]. In a large population database of runners and walkers, a 42.5 decreased risk of brain tumor mortality was seen for those expending ≥1.8 MET-h/day compared to less active individuals [24]. A group of 100 GBM patients receiving inpatient rehabilitation demonstrated nonsignificant difference in survival compared to 312 other GBM patients not receiving rehabilitation, despite the inpatient care recipients' overall lower Karnofsky scores (70 vs 80) at presentation [25]. GBM patients can strengthen with an outpatient exercise program [26]. Walking is reported as the favored form of exercise, with best receptivity to exercise in the post-treatment phase [27]. However, prospectively, adherence and satisfaction is better in supervised rather than unsupervised programs [26].

As with other brain rehabilitation patients, a wide range of management concerns may exist, including *seizures, thromboembolism, headache, fatigue,* and *mood disorders* [18].

Seizures

Seizures are most common in low-grade lesions, and in those involving temporal, frontal, or insular locations, they persist more often after subtotal than total resection [28]. Leviracetam, lamotrigine, and lacosamide are newer antiepileptic agents and are considered first line. Enzyme-inducing agents (carbamazepine, phenytoin, phenobarbital) should be avoided when possible in the setting of chemotherapy [29]. Levetiracetam has no known drug-drug interactions and is popular for prophylaxis. Lacosamide has been shown to be effective as either monotherapy or in combination to reduce seizures in the brain tumor population [30]. Valproic acid, while also shown to be effective, is a CYP450 inhibitor and may potentiate the toxicities of some antineoplastic agents [31].

Thromboembolism

Risk factors for thromboembolism in glioma include older age, three or more comorbidities, leg paresis, glioblastoma multiforme histology, large tumor size, neurosurgery within 61 days, use of chemotherapy, and length of surgery greater than 4 hours [32, 33]. In a study of over 9000 cases of malignant glioma, 715 cases of thromboembolism (7.5%) were found [32]. Another study found a rate of 24% of symptomatic deep venous thrombosis (DVT) in the 17 months following surgery [33]. Low molecular weight heparin is recommended for the first 5–10 days of newly established thromboembolic disease and for long-term secondary prophylaxis for at least 6 months [34]. Risk of intracranial hemorrhage must be considered in patients with active brain metastases.

Headache

In addition to factors causing headaches in the noncancer population, such as hypertension or medications, tumor-related headaches may occur secondary to postoperative pain, increased intracranial pressure, radiation, or chemotherapy [35]. Signs and symptoms in brain tumor patients with headaches that require further evaluation include occurring first thing in the morning or waking the patient at night, progressive, unresponsive to medications, worsening with position change, somnolence, or new neurologic deficits [35]. Acetaminophen is generally the safest medication to treat glioma-associated headaches, with NSAIDs dependent on risk factors and corticosteroids if cerebral edema is present.

Fatigue

Also multifactorial, fatigue is common during cranial radiation and can persist in survivors [36]. See Chap. 2 for more information on cancer-related fatigue.

Mood

Depression and anxiety are the most common mood disorders in glioma patients. Fifteen to twenty percent of glioma patients will be depressed during their illness [37]. Acute mood changes warrant evaluation for delirium. The cause of persistent mood changes is often multifactorial and may be related to impact of the diagnosis, direct effect of tumor, side effects of medications, and comorbid conditions [35]. Maintaining a culture of support and hope is important. Other considerations are the decision-making capacity of the patient, and that anxiety can improve with patients that have received and understand information. Still, patients may vary in their desire for information. For example, some may prefer full information versus a little at a time, or just "critical/important" information [38, 39].

Eye Cancers

Overall, these cancers are rare. The most common is retinoblastoma, which occurs in young children, usually infancy through age five. Retinoblastoma presents with leukocoria (white pupil), strabismus and possible iris color change [40]. Second is melanoma, which is the most common ocular cancer of adulthood, followed by lymphoma. Ocular melanoma represents 5% of all melanomas, and presents with nonspecific visual changes or is diagnosed incidentally [41]. Survival has shown improvement in recent decades, associated with changing trends in treatment towards less reliance on radiation and more on chemotherapy [42]. Fatal metastatic disease, most notably to the liver, develops in up to 50% of patients over 10–25 years [41]. Radiation modalities are the standard of care [43]. Both retinoblastoma and ocular melanoma require lifelong surveillance [40, 43]. The most common tumors to metastasize to the eye are breast and lung cancers, with a predilection for the choroid layer [44]. Table 4.5 outlines the visual effects of ocular or central nervous system neoplasms.

TABLE 4.5 Visual effects of ocular or central nervous system neoplasms

Etiology	Usual presentation	Additional information
Retinoblastoma	Leukocoria (white pupil)	Strabimus if compensating for lack of central vision; iris change in advanced disease
Ocular melanoma	Nonspecific visual changes	May be diagnosed incidentally on routine eye exam
Brain tumor (cerebral)	Varies, blurred or double vision, visual field cut or visual neglect, difficulty recognizing or identifying objects or colors	Meningioma, astrocytomas, metastatic disease, etc.
Brain tumor (posterior fossa)	Double vision	Medulloblastoma; cerebellopontine angle tumors
Brain tumor (optic nerve, sellar, optic chiasm)	Monocular vision loss for tumors affecting the optic nerve(prechiasmal), bitemporal hemionopia for sella turcica lesion, visual field cut in opposite hemifield for optic tract lesion	Pituitary tumors, craniopharyngiomas, neurofibromatosis, suprasellar/optic meningioma

(continued)

TABLE 4.5 (continued)

Etiology	Usual presentation	Additional information
Craniotomy	Limited data; visual field cut reported in 2/400 patient in one series [49]	Surgery is the mainstay of treatment for most tumors
Radiation	Early-conjunctivitis; eyelid edema or erythema; lacrimal gland effects [37] Late-cataract, retinopathy, glaucoma [53] optic neuropathy [20]	Cataract can be addressed more easily than retinopathy or glaucoma Delayed complications dose dependent
Chemotherapy	Systemic: periocular cutaneous and glandular effects (various); ocular surface dryness/sequelae(carmustine, mitomycin); corneal opacities (tamoxifen); cataract (busulfan, methotrexate, toremifene, tamoxifen; corneal toxicity, ocular pain, foreign body sensation, blurred vision, conjunctival hyperemia (cytarabine in combination regimens); glaucoma (interferon alpha); retinopathy (cisplatin; mitotane; tamoxifen; interferon); optic/oculomotor neuropathies (carmustine; vinblastine, vincristine); optic neuropathy (tamoxifen, interferon) [40]	For GBM, most common chemotherapy is temozolamide (headache a more common side effect with this medicine)

Spinal Cord

Intramedullary spinal cord or cauda equina neoplasms are quite rare, comprising 3.1% of all CNS neoplasms, and most malignant spinal cord injuries (SCI) relate to spinal cord compression from bony metastatic disease. Spinal intramedullary lesions include ependymomas, astrocytomas, and hemangioblastomas [45]. The most common presenting feature of malignant SCI is back pain, often worse with recumbent position. The thoracic level is most commonly affected (70%) followed by lumbosacral (20%) and cervical (10%) regions, reflecting the spinal blood supply and thoracic canal diameter.

Tumor types commonly metastasizing to spine include lung, breast, prostate, kidney, and melanoma, and multiple myeloma may also be associated with malignant SCI [46]. Radiation myelitis can also occur. Early recognition has long been recognized as crucial in optimizing chances of maintaining ambulation capacity, though conflicting data exists as to the impact of maintaining ambulatory status on survival, with primary tumor type and Karnofsky performance status being more strongly associated with prognosis [47]. Rapid paralysis and bowel and bladder involvement are relatively poor prognostic functional signs. Motor involvement typically precedes sensory change, with recovery occurring in the reverse order.

The Spine Instability Neoplastic Score (SINS) is a widely used paradigm to assess for the need for operative stabilization [48] (Table 4.6). Surgical stabilization when feasible promotes best outcomes, preserving function and quality of life, and providing symptom relief [5]. Survival is mostly driven by tumor type, with breast and renal cancers more favorable than lung or prostate cancers [5]. The presence of multiple spinal metastases, cervical metastasis, or pathologic fracture had no significant influence on survival. A large international study showed overall survival rates after surgery of 53% at 1 year, 31% at 2 years, and 10% at 5 years, with longer survival in the more recent years of the study period [49].

Individuals with neoplastic SCI have been found to make comparable gains per day in inpatient rehabilitation as traumatic spinal cord patients. Compared to traumatic SCI, typi-

TABLE 4.6 Spine Instability Neoplastic Score (SINS)

Location	
Junctional (occiput-C2, C7-T2, T11-L1, L5-S1)	3
Mobile spine (C3-C6, L2-L4)	2
Semirigid (T3-T10)	1
Rigid (S2-S5)	0
Pain	
Yes	3
Occasional pain but not mechanical	1
Pain-free lesion	0
Bone lesion	
Lytic	2
Mixed	1
Blastic	0
Radiographic spinal alignment	
Subluxation/translation present	4
De novo deformity (kyphosis, scoliosis)	2
Normal alignment	0
Vertebral body collapse	
>50% collapse	3
<50% collapse	2
No collapse with >50% body involved	1
None of the above	0
Posterolateral involvement of spinal elements	
Bilateral	3
Unilateral	1
None of the above	0

From Fisher et al. [49] with permission
Total score: 0–6: stable; 7–12: indeterminate (possibly impending) instability;13–18: high fracture risk. Surgical consultation recommended with total score >7

cally rehabilitation length of stay is shorter, as paraplegia occurs more commonly than tetraplegia, and most cancer-related myelopathy is incomplete [50]. However, the patient with spinal cord neoplasm is typically older than most traumatic SCI-injured patients, with other health comorbidities [51]. As with brain tumor, interrupted stay is more common than with other SCI cases [52]. New et al. [53] outlined a framework for neoplastic SCI rehabilitation, including that acute rehabilitation should be considered when estimated life prognosis is three months or more; they also advised for the rehabilitation team to cultivate a mindset that transfer to a palliative setting or even death should not be viewed as a failure.

Peripheral Polyneuropathy

While peripheral polyneuropathy can occur as a primary effect of tumor, most commonly it is seen as a chemotherapy effect, especially with vinca alkaloids, taxol derivatives, and platinum agents [54] (Table 4.7). Neuropathy may limit the

TABLE 4.7 Chemotherapy-associated polyneuropathy

Agents	Trade name	Nerve fibers	Tumors
Taxanes	Taxol/ Taxotere	Sensory > motor	Breast, lung, ovarian
Platinum	Carboplatin, Oxiplatin	Pure sensory	Lung, ovarian, colon
Cisplatin	Platinol, CDDP	Pure sensory	Lung, ovarian
Thalidomides	Thalomid	Sensory > motor	Myeloma
Vinca alkaloids, Vincristine	Oncovin, Vincasar, others	Motor = sensory	Lymphoma
Immune checkpoint inhibitors	-mab drugs	Demyelination (also myasthenia, myositis)	Advanced disease

extent of chemotherapy able to be delivered. Immune checkpoint inhibitor therapies have been found to produce rare but severe neuromuscular effects including inflammatory neuropathy and myasthenia gravis, and less commonly inflammatory myopathy [55]. Neuropathy presentation may precede the cancer diagnosis. Treatment includes medications for neuropathic pain (anticonvulsants, antidepressants), nonconstrictive footwear, orthotics, assistive and adaptive devices, and fall prevention. Radiation therapy can produce peripheral nerve lesions, including brachial plexopathy or lumbosacral plexopathy [56]. (See Radiation Fibrosis chapter for further information.)

Case

A 58-year-old woman with history of hypertension, hyperlipidemia, hypothyroidism, prediabetes, obesity, gastroesophageal reflux disease, and low back pain presented to the emergency department with falls and altered mental status. MRI showed right frontal brain mass, for which she underwent elective subtotal resection 11 days later. Pathology revealed atypical meningothelial meningioma, WHO grade II. Her acute course was notable for hyponatremia. She received a seven-day course of levetiracetamfor seizure prophylaxis and was transferred to acute rehabilitation on dexamethasone taper. Her functional status improved.

Five weeks after her surgery, the patient began radiation therapy with 5600 cGy provided over 5 weeks. The patient was seen for her initial outpatient physiatry appointment shortly before the start of radiation therapy, and began outpatient physical, occupational and speech therapies. Major symptoms included fatigue, bilateral knee pain, low mood, amotivation, difficulty with memory and cognitive focusing, and intermittent headache. She expressed desire to return to work as soon as possible. Outpatient therapy was tolerated though marked by missed appointments, including transportation barriers. Two months later she had completed radiation, and was off corticosteroids.

This case illustrates multiple issues. Meningioma is usually benign, but may have a malignant variant. Her course was complicated by cerebral edema, due to radiation encephalopathy versus residual effect of tumor, most likely the former. While early corticosteroid wean can be considered desirable, in this case prolonged treatment was required. Through all of this, return to work remained an important focus for this patient, as it should to the care team, if appropriate.

Multiple Choice Questions

1. Which is the most common segment for spinal cord injury due to neoplasm?

   A. Cervical
   B. Thoracic
   C. Lumbar
   D. Sacral

2. Which tumor type is most likely to be associated with a paraneoplastic peripheral polyneuropathy?

   A. Small cell lung cancer
   B. Prostate cancer
   C. Breast cancer
   D. Squamous cell head and neck cancer

3. Which of the following is true, in general, of patients with central nervous system malignancies receiving acute rehabilitation?

   A. Interrupted stay occurs less frequently than with other noncancer neurorehabilitation patients.
   B. Functional outcomes as measured by FIM efficiency are similar to noncancer neurorehabilitation patients.
   C. Length of stay is longer than noncancer neurorehabilitation patients.
   D. Individuals with brain metastatic disease have worse FIM scores than other brain tumor patients.

4. What is the most common presenting feature of spinal cord neoplasm?

   A. Sensory loss
   B. Bladder incontinence
   C. Falls
   D. Back pain

5. In comparing pediatric and adult brain tumor populations, which of the following is true?

   A. Incidence of malignant brain tumor is higher in children than in adults.
   B. Long-term survival is better for most pediatric tumor types compared to most adult primary brain malignancies.
   C. Young children are less likely to experience long-term cognitive sequelae of whole brain radiation than are young adults.
   D. Adult primary brain tumor types are more likely to involve the posterior fossa.

Answers

1. B
2. A
3. B
4. D
5. B

References

1. Noone AM, Howlader N, Krapcho M, Miller D, Brest A, Yu M, Ruhl J, Tatalovich Z, Mariotto A, Lewis DR, Chen HS, Feuer EJ, Cronin KA, editors. Cancer stat facts: brain and other nervous system cancer. In: SEER cancer statistics review, 1975–2015, National Cancer Institute, Bethesda, https://seer.cancer.gov/csr/1975_2015/, based on Nov 2017 SEER data submission, posted to the SEER web site, Apr 2018.

2. Ostrom QT, Gittleman H, Truitt G, et al. CBTRUS statistical report: primary brain and other central nervous system tumors diagnosed in the United States in 2011–2015. Neuro-Oncology. 2018;20(S4):1–86.
3. Cagney DN, Martin AM, Catalano PJ, et al. Incidence and prognosis of patients with brain metastases at diagnosis of systemic malignancy: a population-based study. Neuro-Oncology. 2017;19(11):1511–21.
4. Achrol AS, Rennert RC, Anders C, et al. Brain metastases. Nat Rev Dis Primers. 2019;5(1):5.
5. Yao A, Sarkiss CA, Ladner TR, Jenkins AL. Contemporary spinal oncology treatment paradigms and outcomes for metastatic tumors to the spine: a systematic review of breast, prostate, renal, and lung metastases. J Clin Neurosci. 2017;41:11–23.
6. National Collaborating Centre for Cancer (UK). Metastatic spinal cord compression. Diagnosis and management of patients at risk of or with metastatic spinal cord compression. NICE clinical guidelines, no. 75. Cardiff: National Collaborating Centre for Cancer (UK); 2008, ISBN-13: 978-0-9558265-1-1.
7. Lehmann J, DeLisa JA, Warren CG, et al. Cancer rehabilitation assessment of need development and education of a model of care. Arch Phys Med Rehabil. 1978;59:410–9.
8. Mukand JA, Blackinton DD, Crincolli MG, et al. Incidence of neurologic deficits and rehabilitation of patients with brain tumors. Am J Phys Med Rehabil. 2001;80:346–50.
9. Lustig RH, Post SR, Srivannaboon K, et al. Risk factors for the development of obesity in children surviving brain tumors. J Clin Endocrinol Metab. 2003;88(2):611–6.
10. Short PF, Vasey JJ, Tunceli K. Employment pathways in a large cohort of adult cancer survivors. Cancer. 2005;103:1292–301.
11. Ellenberg L, Liu Q, Gioia G, et al. Neurocognitive status in long-term survivors of childhood CNS malignancies: a report from the Childhood Cancer Survivor Study. Neuropsychology. 2009;23(6):705–17.
12. Lonjaret L, Guyonnet M, Berard E, et al. Postoperative complications after craniotomy for brain tumor surgery. Anaesth Crit Care Pain Med. 2017;36:213–8.
13. Sawaya R, Hammoud M, Schoppa D, et al. Neurosurgical outcomes in a modern series of 400 craniotomies for treatment of parenchymal tumors. Neurosurgery. 1998;42(5):1044–55.
14. Sharpar S, Mhatre PV, Huang ME. Update on brain tumors: new developments in neuro-oncologic diagnosis and treatment, and impact on rehabilitation strategies. PM R. 2016;8:678–89.

15. Dropcho EJ. Neurotoxicity of radiation therapy. Neurol Clin. 2010;28:217–34.
16. Greene-Schloesser D, Robbins ME, Peiffer AM, et al. Radiation-induced brain injury: a review. Front Oncol. 2012;2:1–18.
17. Dietrich J, Rao K, Pastorino S, Kesari S. Corticosteroids in brain cancer patients: benefits and pitfalls. Expert Rev Clin Pharmacol. 2011;4(2):233–42.
18. Vargo M. Brain tumors and metastases. Phys Med Rehabil Clin N Am. 2017;28:115–41.
19. Marciniak CM, Sliwa JA, Heinemann AW, Semik PE. Functional outcomes of persons with brain tumors after inpatient rehabilitation. Arch Phys Med Rehabil. 2001;82:457–63.
20. Khan F, Amatya B, Drummond K, et al. Effectiveness of integrated multidisciplinary rehabilitation in primary brain cancer survivors in an Australian community cohort: a controlled clinical trial. J Rehabil Med. 2014;46:754–60.
21. McCarty S, Keeshin S, Eickmeyer SM, et al. Evaluation of the cost of comprehensive outpatient therapies in patients with malignant brain tumors. Am J Phys Med Rehabil. 2017;96:341–6.
22. Langenbahn DM, Ashman T, Cantor J, et al. An evidence-based review of cognitive rehabilitation in medical conditions affecting cognitive function. Arch Phys Med Rehabil. 2013;94:271–86.
23. Ruden E, Reardon DA, Coan AD, et al. Exercise behavior, functional capacity, and survival in adults with malignant recurrent glioma. J Clin Oncol. 2011;29:2918–23.
24. Williams PT. Reduced risk of brain cancer mortality from walking and running. Med Sci Sports Exerc. 2014;46(5):927–32.
25. Roberts PS, Nuño M, Sherman D, et al. The impact of inpatient rehabilitation on function and survival of newly diagnosed patients with glioblastoma. PM R. 2014;6:514–21.
26. Hansen A, Søgaard K, Minet LR, Jarden JO. A 12-week interdisciplinary rehabilitation trial in patients with gliomas – a feasibility study. Disabil Rehabil. 2018;40(12):1379–85.
27. Jones LW, Guill B, Keir ST. Exercise interest and preferences among patients diagnosed with primary brain cancer. Support Care Cancer. 2007;15:47–55.
28. Englot DJ, Chang EF, Vecht CJ. Epilepsy and brain tumors. Handb Clin Neurol. 2016;134:267–85.
29. Vecht CJ, van Breemen M. Optimizing therapy of seizures in patients with brain tumors. Neurology. 2006;67(Suppl 4):S10–3.

30. Benit CP, Kerkhof M, Duran-Peña A, Vecht CJ. Seizures as complications in cancer. In: Cancer neurology in clinical practice. Cham: Springer; 2018. p. 153–69.
31. Bourg V, Lebrun C, Chichmanian RM, Thomas P, Frenay M. Nitroso-urea-cisplatin-based chemotherapy associated with valproate: increase of haematologic toxicity. Ann Oncol. 2001;12(2):217–9.
32. Semrad TJ, O'Donnell R, Wun T, Chew H, Harvey D, Zhou H, White RH. Epidemiology of venous thromboembolism in 9489 patients with malignant glioma. J Neurosurg. 2007;106(4):601–8.
33. Marras LC, Geerts WH, Perry JR. The risk of venous thromboembolism is increased throughout the course of malignant glioma: an evidence-based review. Cancer. 2000;89(3):640–6.
34. Lyman GH, Bohlke K, Khorana AA, Kuderer NM, Lee AY, Arcelus JI, Balaban EP, Clarke JM, Flowers CR, Francis CW, Gates LE. Venous thromboembolism prophylaxis and treatment in patients with cancer: American Society of Clinical Oncology clinical practice guideline update 2014. J Clin Oncol. 2015;33(6):654.
35. Siegel C, Armstrong TS. Nursing guide to management of major symptoms in patients with malignant glioma. Seminars in oncology nursing. 2018; 34(5):513–27.
36. Armstrong TS, Cron SG, Bolanos EV, Gilbert MR, Kang DH. Risk factors for fatigue severity in primary brain tumor patients. Cancer. 2010;116:2707–15.
37. Rooney AG, Brown PD, Reijneveld JC, Grant R. Depression in glioma: a primer for clinicians and researchers. J Neurol Neurosurg Psychiatry. 2014;85:230–5.
38. Salander P, Bergenheim T, Henriksson R. The creation of protection and hope in patients with malignant brain tumours. Soc Sci Med. 1996;42(7):985–96.
39. Vargo M, Henriksson R, Salander P. Rehabilitation of patients with glioma. Handb Clin Neurol. 2016;134:287–304.
40. Dimaras H, Corson TW, Cobrinik D, et al. Retinoblastoma. Nat Rev Dis Primers. 2015;1:15021. https://doi.org/10.1038/nrdp.2015.21.
41. Amaro A, Gangemi R, Piaggio F, et al. The biology of uveal melanoma. Cancer Metastasis Rev. 2017;36:109–40.
42. Singh M, Durairaj P, Yeung J. Uveal melanoma: a review of the literature. Oncol Ther. 2018;6:87–10.4.

43. Mishra KK, Chiu-Tsao ST, Orton CG. Particle therapy is ideal for the treatment of ocular melanomas. Point counterpoint. Med Phys. 2016;43(2):631–4.
44. Rundle P (2017) Photodynamic therapy for eye cancer. Biomedicine 5(4) pii E69; doi:https://doi.org/10.3390/biomedicines5040069.
45. Samartzis D, Gillis CC, Shih P, et al. Intramedullary spinal cord tumors: part i—epidemiology, pathophysiology, and diagnosis. Global Spine J. 2015;5:425–35.
46. Byrne TN. Spinal cord compression from epidural metastases. NEJM. 1992;327:614–9.
47. Barcena A, et al. Spinal metastatic disease. An analysis of factors determining functional prognosis and the choice of treatment. Neurosurgery. 1984;15:820–7.
48. Feng JT, Yang XG, Wang F, et al. Prognostic discrepancy on overall survival between ambulatory and nonambulatory patients with metastatic spinal cord compression. World Neurosurg. 2019;121:e322–32.
49. Fisher CG, DiPaola CP, Ryken TC, et al. A novel classification system for spinal instability in neoplastic disease: an evidence-based approach and expert consensus from the Spine Oncology Study Group. Spine. 2010;35:E1221–9.
50. Wright E, Ricciardi F, Arts M, et al. Metastatic spine tumor epidemiology: comparison of trends in surgery across two decades and three continents. World Neurosurg. 2018;114:e809–17.
51. McKinley WO, Huang E, Brunsvold KT. Neoplastic vs traumatic spinal cord injury: an outcome comparison after acute rehabilitation. Arch Phys Med Rehabil. 1999;80(10):1253–7.
52. Alam E, Wilson RD, Vargo M. Inpatient cancer rehabilitation: a retrospective comparison of transfer back to acute care between patients with neoplasm and other rehabilitation patients. Arch Phys Med Rehabil. 2008;89(7):1284–9.
53. New PW, Marshall R, Stubblefield MD, Scivoletto G. Rehabilitation of people with spinal cord damage due to tumor: literature review, international survey and practical recommendations for optimizing their rehabilitation. J Spinal Cord Med. 2017;40(2):213–21.
54. Hausheer FH, Schilsky RL, Bain S, et al. Diagnosis, management and evaluation of chemotherapy induced peripheral neuropathy. Semin Oncol. 2006;33(1):15–49.

55. Kolb NA, Trevino CR, Waheed W, et al. Neuromuscular complications of immune checkpoint inhibitor therapy. Muscle Nerve.
2018;58:10–22.
56. Harper CM, Thomas JE, Cascino TL, Litchy WJ. Distinction
between neoplastic and radiation-induced brachial plexopathy,
with emphasis on the role of EMG. Neurology. 1989;39(4):502–6.

Chapter 5
Cancer of the Urinary Tract and Genital Organs: Female and Male

Michael Fediw and Sean Smith

Prostate Cancer

Overview and Oncologic Treatments

Prostate cancer is the most common cancer among male patients and represents close to 10% of new cancer cases in the USA annually. Despite it's high prevalence, prostate cancer has a 5-year survival rate of 98.2% and accounts for only 4.8% of all cancer deaths annually. The treatment for prostate cancer, however, may lead to pain, weakness, incontinence, and other impairments, of which physiatrists and other rehabilitation providers should be aware.

Treatment for prostate cancer may include systemic therapy, radiation, and/or surgery. Generally, prostate cancer is divided into castration-sensitive and castration-resistant subgroups based on response to decreasing levels of circulating androgens. Systemic therapies may include androgen deprivation therapy (ADT), chemotherapy, immunotherapy, mitoxantrone, ketoconazole, or other agents. Table 5.1 describes

M. Fediw (✉) · S. Smith
University of Michigan, Department of Physical Medicine and Rehabilitation, Ann Arbor, MI, USA

© Springer Nature Switzerland AG 2020
J. Baima, A. Khanna (eds.), *Cancer Rehabilitation*,
https://doi.org/10.1007/978-3-030-44462-4_5

TABLE 5.1 Agents used in prostate cancer and their toxicities

Common treatments	Toxicities
Androgen receptor pathway blocker (Enzalutamide)	Metabolic disturbance, musculoskeletal pain, flushing
Tyrosine kinase inhibitor (Cabozantinib)	Heavy bleeding, altered taste, weight loss
Androgen biosynthesis inhibitor (Abiraterone)	Gastrointestinal issues, metabolic disturbance, hypertension, elevated liver enzymes, joint and muscle aches
[a]PD-1 inhibitors (Pembrolizumab, Nivolumab)	Arthralgia, pancytopenia, nausea, elevated liver function tests (LFTs)

[a]PD-1 inhibitors are newer treatments with clinical trials ongoing for efficacy

some common treatments and their potential toxicities in the treatment of prostate cancer.

Radiation often involves either brachytherapy – wherein radioactive implants are inserted into prostatic tissue – or more traditional external beam radiation therapy to the prostate and surrounding tissue. Acutely, radiation can cause pain and swelling, in addition to proctitis, fatigue, and skin breakdown. Long term, radiation can cause fibrosis of muscles and ligaments leading to weakness, pain, incontinence, and potentially lumbosacral plexus damage.

Surgery may also be indicated for a patient, and carries with it high risks of pelvic floor dysfunction, erectile dysfunction, and pain.

Musculoskeletal Implications of Treatment

Androgen deprivation therapy is a hallmark of prostate cancer treatment and involves reducing testosterone availability through receptor blockade and/or decreased production. The side effects of ADT can be quite detrimental to physical function. As a result of ADT, mesenchymal stem cells are diverted from myogenic to lipogenic pathways, commonly leading to sarcopenic obesity and weight gain. Metabolic syndrome and increased insulin resistance may also occur. As muscle weakness develops, patients may develop painful tendinopathies, mechanical joint pain, and myofascial pain.

Resistance and aerobic exercise have been shown to help mitigate these changes in body composition without increasing PSA or testosterone [1]. Alibhai et al. conducted a small randomized controlled trial (RCT) of different exercise programs on men with prostate cancer receiving ADT, which suggested that one-on-one exercise training compared to group exercise had comparable improvements in quality of life and fitness [2]. Additionally, supervised exercise programs had increased compliance compared to a self-reported exercise regimen.

Decreased bone mineral density is another side effect of ADT that may be underestimated on Dual-Energy X-ray Absorptiometry (DEXA) scans in this population [3]. Weakening of bone places patients at increased risk for fractures, with male patients experiencing higher rates of mortality with osteoporotic fractures compared to women [4]. Bisphosphonates, denosumab, selective estrogen receptor modulators (SERMS), calcium supplementation, and vitamin D supplementation may all be used to prevent and treat bone density loss. A randomized placebo controlled trial of men with castration-resistant prostate cancer receiving zoledronic acid demonstrated an 11% decrease in experiencing a skeletal-related event (SRE), prolonged median time to first SRE, and a 36% reduction in ongoing risk of SRE compared to placebo [5].

In addition to pharmacologic management of bone density loss, resistance-based exercise should be prescribed to patients after a physician evaluation. If patients do not have significant balance impairment and are not at risk for fracture from metastatic disease, an individually tailored strength training program should be recommended and has been shown to improve bone mineral density in the lumbar spine and femoral heads

[6, 7]. Furthermore, Kukuljian et al. found that progressive resistance training with vitamin D supplementation improved bone mineral density by 1.5% in the lumbar spine and 0.7% in the femoral head in older men with osteopenia [8].

Evaluation and Management of Bone Metastases

Prostate cancer has a high affinity for metastasizing to bone and is unique in that it characteristically produces osteoblastic bone lesions, although osteolytic lesions may also occur [9]. Despite osteoblastic lesions being more dense, they are structurally weaker than normal bone and thus more susceptible to fracture [10]. Spinal metastases may lead to catastrophic effects from spinal cord compromise, either from epidural disease or pathologic vertebral fracture compressing the cord. Patients with spinal cord injury should be rehabilitated through the standard of care [11], which is beyond the scope of this chapter. For patients with spinal metastases of unclear stability, the Spine Instability Neoplastic Score (SINS) criteria may be used to determine stability of spinal metastases [12]. The scale evaluates vertebral stability based on spinal location of tumor, presence of mechanical pain, bone lesion type (osteoblastic versus osteolytic), spinal alignment, vertebral body collapse, and posterior spinal involvement and classifies vertebral columns as low, intermediate, and at high risk of instability.

In patients with stable vertebral metastatic disease, rehabilitation interventions for mechanical pain should focus on core strengthening without significant flexion and twisting of the spine. Additionally, interventional pain procedures such as epidural steroid injections and medial branch blocks should be considered in patients with compressive radiculopathies and symptomatic spondylosis, respectively.

For long bone metastases, the authors recommend Mirels' criteria to assess stability. It evaluates stability based on location of tumor, pain, bone lesion quality, and size of lesion relative to bony diameter to help determine the need for surgical fixation. A Mirels' score less than eight is considered safe to irradiate with minimal risk of fracture [13]. For stable lesions, rehabilitation interventions should focus on strengthening surrounding musculature and improving bone density. Providers should have a low threshold for ordering imaging studies in the presence of worsening pain, as metastatic lesions may have progressed.

Multimodal exercise can improve overall physical function in patients with a history of prostate cancer, even those with advanced disease. Galvao et al. found that a supervised program of flexibility, resistance training, and aerobic conditioning in men with prostate cancer metastatic to the bone improved patient-reported physical functioning and lower extremity strength compared to a control group who did not receive additional exercise interventions [14]. Additionally, there were no fractures or adverse events in this study of over 50 men, suggesting that exercise is safe when prescribed by a physician who evaluates the patient before beginning a program.

Pelvic Floor Dysfunction

Pelvic floor dysfunction with erectile dysfunction frequently occurs after surgery or radiation for prostate cancer, with urinary and bowel incontinence being the most common side effects [15]. However, the rates of men experiencing some or all of these symptoms can vary based on the type of treatment [16]. These symptoms can be particularly distressing and may be associated with decreased quality of life and satisfaction with treatment outcome [17].

A recent systematic review by Goonewardene et al. found that biofeedback and presurgical and postsurgical pelvic floor exercises improved urinary incontinence and erectile dysfunction after radical prostatectomy [18]. Exercises that focus on improving deep and superficial pelvic floor muscle strengthening, neuromuscular re-education, and behavior modification techniques seem to be most effective, and patients should be considered for these interventions when they report symptoms of pelvic/perineal pain, incontinence, or erectile dysfunction [19].

Pelvic floor exercises are helpful even before a prostatectomy. Goonewardene et al. found that preoperative pelvic floor strengthening improved continence postoperatively, particularly if exercises were continued after recovery from surgery [18]. In that systematic review, the authors concluded that all patients undergoing a radical prostatectomy should "exercise their pelvic floor muscles to maintain normal pelvic floor function and start prior to surgery." This underscores the point that comprehensive rehabilitation in pelvic floor dysfunction should include at least education preoperatively, and that prehabilitation has a role in preventing pelvic floor dysfunction.

In addition to pelvic rehabilitation, interventional procedures may help with treatment of cancer-associated pain in men with prostate cancer. Innervation of the pelvis, pelvic viscera, internal and external genitalia, anus, and coccyx is through sympathetic mediated pathways of the superior hypogastric plexus, ganglion impar, and pudendal nerve [20]. The ganglion impar generally can transmit pelvic pain below the umbilicus, whereas unilateral and/or penile/vaginal pain may be generated by the pudendal nerve. A thorough history and physical exam may help identify the region and nerve causing the symptoms. Blockade of these structures has been described for the treatment of pain from various pain generators in the pelvis [20–22]. Physicians should be aware of these procedures as potential options to treat pain of the pelvic organs, genitalia, perineum, and coccyx.

Gynecologic Cancer

Overview and Oncologic Treatment

Gynecologic cancer is a general term for a group of cancers that include uterine, ovarian, cervical, vaginal, and vulvar cancers. Uterine cancer, more specifically endometrial cancer, is by far the most common gynecologic cancer followed by ovarian, cervical, vaginal, and vulvar cancer, respectively [23]. The effects of gynecologic cancer and its treatment can be quite impairing, as Hammer et al. reported that 53% of women diagnosed with uterine cancer are unable to participate fully in the activities that they wish to [24]. Despite being significantly less common than other gynecologic malignancies, ovarian cancer accounts for the most deaths of gynecologic cancers due to often being in advanced stage at time of diagnosis. This section will focus on the common toxicities and functional impairments related to the treatment of gynecologic cancers such as pelvic floor dysfunction, pelvic and lower extremity lymphedema, aromatase-inhibitor-induced arthralgia, and chemotherapy-induced peripheral neuropathy (Table 5.2).

TABLE 5.2 Agents used in gynecologic cancers and their toxicities

Common treatments	Common toxicities
Platinum agents (cisplatin, carboplatin, oxaliplatin)	Nausea, alopecia, renal impairment, ototoxicity, neuropathy, PRES
Taxanes (docetaxel, paclitaxel)	Pancytopenia, alopecia, neuropathy, arthralgia, myalgia, nausea, renal impairment
VEG-F inhibitor (bevacizumab)	Fatigue, nausea, arthralgia, bleeding, muscular weakness, neuropathy, HTN, GI upset
Gemcitabine	Elevated liver enzymes, nausea,
Topoisomerase inhibitors (irinotecan, topotecan)	Pancytopenia, elevated liver enzymes, GI upset, asthenia, alopecia, mucositis, rash
[a]Pembrolizumab	Decreased appetite, arthralgia, pancytopenia, nausea, electrolyte disturbance

Key: *VEG-F* vascular endothelial growth factor, *PRES* posterior reversible leukoencephalopathy syndrome, HTN hypertension
[a]PD-1 inhibitors are newer therapies with clinical trials ongoing to prove efficacy

Pelvic and Lower Extremity Lymphedema

Pelvic and lower extremity lymphedema is a common comorbidity in gynecologic cancer resulting from tumor invasion of the lymphatics, lymph node dissection, or radiation. Lymphedema can lead to pain, impaired mobility and activities of daily living, psychological distress, social isolation, and decreased quality of life. Biglia et al. reported in a systematic review of primary studies on women with lower extremity lymphedema from gynecologic cancers that the incidence of lower extremity lymphedema, while variable, was as high as 47%, 59.1%, and 40.8% in endometrial, cervical, and ovarian cancers, respectively [25]. Of all gynecologic malignancies, patients treated for vulvar cancer have the highest rate of lower extremity lymphedema, with ovarian being the lowest [26]. Obesity, number of lymph nodes surgically removed, history of chemotherapy, history of radiation therapy, premorbid nonsteroidal anti-inflammatory analgesic use, and presence of infection are all independent risk factors for the development of lymphedema [27].

Lymphedema is usually a clinical diagnosis that is made by a provider knowledgeable about lymphedema. The International Society of Lymphology (ISL) categorizes lymphedema into four stages. These stages range from 0 to 3 with a higher number associated with more severe edema [28] (Table 5.3).

Sometimes, it is not clear if edema is lymphatic in origin (lymphedema) or if there is another cause for swelling, such as venous insufficiency, mechanical compression of vasculature (as would be seen with tumor recurrence), deep venous thrombosis, cardiac and/or renal failure, neurogenic edema, or lipedema. In these cases, further testing such as venous duplex scans to evaluate for valve integrity, lymphoscintigraphy, and/or imaging to rule out compression may be necessary.

Complete Decongestive Therapy (CDT) is the gold standard for lymphedema management. It consists of two phases of treatment. The initial, decongestive phase utilizes skin care,

TABLE 5.3 International society of lymphology stages of lymphedema [28]

Stage 0	Subclinical stage where lymph transport is disrupted but swelling has not yet occurred. May have subjective symptoms.
Stage 1	Swelling of fluid that is high in protein content. Swelling reduces with limb elevation. Pitting may occur.
Stage 2	Swelling that rarely reduces with limb elevation alone. Pitting is manifest early on but may decrease later in this stage as excess subcutaneous fat and fibrosis develop.
Stage 3	Trophic skin changes with thickening, acanthosis, worsening of fat deposition and fibrosis, and warty overgrowth. Elephantiasis.

manual lymphatic drainage (MLD), and compression bandages to reduce extremity volume. The second, maintenance phase utilizes continued skin care, MLD and compressions stockings to maintain reduced limb size. Intermittent pneumatic compression may also be used in the maintenance phase [29]. A pilot study by Do et al. in endometrial, cervical, and ovarian cancer patients with lymphedema after cancer-related surgery undergoing CDT with a comprehensive rehab program vs. CDT alone found that strength, physical function, and fatigue were improved without adversely affecting lymphedema status when a comprehensive rehab program (stretching, strengthening, and aerobic exercise) was performed in conjunction with CDT [30]. Physicians should be aware of the indications for referring to CDT, which should ideally be performed by a therapist with advanced training to treat the condition.

Aromatase-Inhibitor-Induced Arthralgia

Despite the prevalence of estrogen receptor and progestin receptor expression throughout the female reproductive tract and in gynecologic tumors, use of selective estrogen receptor modulators (SERMs) and aromatase inhibitors (AIs) has only shown to be efficacious in small subpopulations of gynecologic cancers [31], often those of endometrial origin. Data on aromatase-inhibitor-induced arthralgia is lacking in the gynecologic cancer population, but has been well described in patients undergoing AI therapy for breast cancer. Rehabilitation physicians should be aware of use of hormonal therapy in gynecologic cancer survivors and its potential to cause joint pain and loss of function. See Breast Cancer chapter for more details.

Chemotherapy-Induced Peripheral Neuropathy

Chemotherapy regimens for gynecologic cancers frequently include platinum-based agents and taxane-based chemotherapy, which are associated with neurotoxicity causing peripheral neuropathy. Patients receiving these agents may experience numbness, tingling, pain, weakness, and balance impairment. In patients who receive these chemotherapy types and who develop new-onset symmetric, distal sensory changes, clinicians should perform a thorough neurologic evaluation including gait assessment to diagnose and subsequently manage the symptoms of chemotherapy-induced peripheral neuropathy. If it is unclear whether the patient has developed these symptoms, nerve conduction studies may be helpful. Management is multimodal, and often includes a combination of pain management with oral analgesia and desensitization modalities, gait and balance training, orthotic use, and fall-risk education.

Pelvic Floor Dysfunction

Pelvic floor dysfunction (PFD) has a high prevalence in the gynecologic cancer population and includes urinary, bowel, and sexual dysfunction. Reported rates of PFD vary amongst different gynecologic cancer types and treatments. Limited data exists comparing the prevalence of PFD in gynecologic cancers to the general population [32].

Pelvic floor therapy, which typically involves a combination of strengthening weak muscles and stretching/releasing tight antagonist muscles, has been shown to be an effective treatment of PFD in the general population [33]. Evidence to date has shown promise for pelvic floor therapy for PFD in the gynecologic cancer population as well. A pilot study by Yang et al. in predominantly cervical cancer survivors found that a pelvic floor rehabilitation program improved pelvic floor strength, sexual desire, sexual function, pain, and physical function compared to a control group [34]. Rutledge et al. also demonstrated that urinary incontinence in gynecologic cancer patients improved with a combination of pelvic floor exercises and behavioral training compared to a control group [35].

Renal Cancer

Kidney cancer is a common cancer, ranking in the top 10 for both men and women with close to 90% of these being renal cell carcinoma (RCC). Kidney cancer carries a generally favorable prognosis with 75% 5-year survival rate across all stages. This number increases to 93% with disease that is localized. This section will identify two key rehabilitation needs in this population, though as with all cancer survivors, those treated for RCC may develop impairments based on how advanced their disease is and the oncologic treatment rendered (Table 5.4).

Sarcopenia is a common problem in renal cell carcinoma and is an independent predictor of overall survival [36]. Additionally, sarcopenia has been associated with targeted therapies for renal cell carcinoma, particularly tyrosine kinase inhibitors targeting the Vascular Endothelial Growth Factor (VEGF) and Mammalian Target of Rapamycin (mTOR) pathways [37]. There is limited data looking at the impact of rehabilitation and exercise on the effects of sarcopenia in RCC. Monfardini et al. reported that in patients with genitourinary cancers, including RCC, only 25% of

TABLE 5.4 Agents used in renal cancer and their toxicities

Common treatments	Common toxicities
Tyrosine kinase inhibitors (axitinib, pazopanib, sorafenib, sunitinib)	HTN, nausea, asthenia, bleeding, arthralgia, elevated liver enzymes, electrolyte disturbance, cardiac dysfunction
CTLA-4 inhibitor (Ipilimumab)	Fatigue, pruritis, dermatitis, rash, colitis
PD-1 inhibitor (Nivolumab)	Elevated liver enzymes, electrolyte disturbance, rash, musculoskeletal pain, nausea
VEGF inhibitor (Bevacizumab)	

Key: *CTLA-4* human cytotoxic T-lymphcyte antigen 4, *PD-1* programmed cell death-1 protein, *VEG-F* vascular endothelial growth factor

patients experiencing difficulty with ADLs and 10% of patients experiencing difficulty with IADLs were being referred for rehabilitation. This suggests that functional needs and muscle loss may be overlooked in patients with RCC. Shmid et al. found that moderate to vigorous activity was associated with decreased mortality in RCC patients. A small pilot study by Rosenberger showed that a machine-based resistance program was feasible, safe, and increased strength in patients with RCC. This would suggest that a guided exercise plan should be incorporated into the treatment of patients with RCC.

A common site of RCC metastases is the bony spine. Lipton et al. showed that Zoledronic acid decreases the risk of skeletal-related events in patients with metastatic RCC. Conventional radiotherapy has traditionally been associated with poor control of spinal metastases from RCC, but more recent development of stereotactic radiosurgery (SRS) has resulted in improved treatment of spinal disease and painful metastases. While SRS has improved pain and local control of spinal metastases, vertebral compression fracture after SRS has been reported to be 16–27.5% [38].

This underscores the need for providers to discuss spinal precautions with patients who have vertebral metastases regardless of pain.

References

1. Cormie P, Zopf EM. Exercise medicine for the management of androgen deprivation therapy-related side effects in prostate cancer. Urol Oncol. 2018. pii: S1078-1439(18)30390-9. https://doi.org/10.1016/j.urolonc.2018.10.008. [Epub ahead of print].
2. Alibhai SMH, Santa Mina D, Ritvo P, Tomlinson G, Sabiston C, Krahn M, Durbano S, Matthew A, Warde P, O'Neill M, Timilshina N, Segal R, Culos-Reed N. A phase II randomized controlled trial of three exercise delivery methods in men with prostate cancer on androgen deprivation therapy. BMC Cancer. 2019;19(1):2. https://doi.org/10.1186/s12885-018-5189-5.
3. Russell N, Grossmann M.Management of bone and metabolic effects of androgen deprivation therapy. Urol Oncol. 2018. pii: S1078-1439(18)30389-2. https://doi.org/10.1016/j.urolonc.2018.10.007. [Epub ahead of print].
4. Kessler ER. Management of metastatic prostate cancer in frail/elderly patients. Oncology (Williston Park). 2018;32(11):570–3.
5. Saad F, Gleason DM, Murray R, Tchekmedyian S, Venner P, Lacombe L, et al. Long-term efficacy of zoledronic acid for the prevention of skeletal complications in patients with metastatic hormone-refractory prostate cancer. J Natl Cancer Inst. 2004;96:879–82.
6. McMillan L, Zengin A, Ebeling P, Scott D. Prescribing physical activity for the prevention and treatment of osteoporosis in older adults. Healthcare. 2017;5(4):85. Multidisciplinary Digital Publishing Institute.
7. Whiteford J, Ackland TR, Dhaliwal SS, James AP, Woodhouse JJ, Price R, Prince RL, Kerr DA. Effects of a 1-year randomized controlled trial of resistance training on lower limb bone and muscle structure and function in older men. Osteoporos Int. 2010;21(9):1529–36.
8. Kukuljan S, Nowson CA, Bass SL, Sanders K, Nicholson GC, Seibel MJ, Salmon J, Daly RM. Effects of a multi-component exercise program and calcium–vitamin-D 3-fortified milk on bone mineral density in older men: a randomised controlled trial. Osteoporos Int. 2009;20(7):1241–51.

9. Logothetis CJ, Lin SH. Osteoblasts in prostate cancer metastasis to bone. Nat Rev Cancer. 2005;5(1):21–8.
10. Lin SC, Yu-Lee LY, Lin SH. Osteoblastic factors in prostate cancer bone metastasis. Curr Osteoporos Rep. 2018;16(6):642–7. https://doi.org/10.1007/s11914-018-0480-6. Review
11. Ruppert LM. Malignant spinal cord compression: adapting conventional rehabilitation approaches. Phys Med Rehabil Clin. 2017;28(1):101–14.
12. Fisher CG, DiPaola CP, Ryken TC, Bilsky MH, Shaffrey CI, Berven SH, Harrop JS, Fehlings MG, Boriani S, Chou D, Schmidt MH, Polly DW, Biagini R, Burch S, Dekutoski MB, Ganju A, Gerszten PC, Gokaslan ZL, Groff MW, Liebsch NJ, Mendel E, Okuno SH, Patel S, Rhines LD, Rose PS, Sciubba DM, Sundaresan N, Tomita K, Varga PP, Vialle LR, Vrionis FD, Yamada Y, Fourney DR. A novel classification system for spinal instability in neoplastic disease. Spine (Phila Pa 1976). 2010;35(22):E1221–9. https://doi.org/10.1097/BRS.0b013e3181e16ae2.
13. Mirels H. Metastatic disease in long bones: a proposed scoring system for diagnosing impending pathologic fractures. Clin Orthop Relat Res. 1989;(415 Suppl):S4–13.
14. Galvao DA, Taaffe DR, Spry N, Cormie P, Joseph D, Chambers SK, Chee R, Peddle-Mcintyre CJ, Hart NH, Baumann FT, Denham J. Exercise preserves physical function in prostate cancer patients with bone metastases. Med Sci Sports Exerc. 2018;50(3):393.
15. Anderson CA, Omar MI, Campbell SE, Hunter KF, Cody JD, Glazener C. Conservative management for postprostatectomy urinary incontinence. Cochrane Database Syst Rev. 2015;1:17.
16. Jang JW, Drumm MR, Efstathiou JA, Paly JJ, Niemierko A, Ancukiewicz M, Talcott JA, Clark JA, Zietman AL. Long-term quality of life after definitive treatment for prostate cancer: patient-reported outcomes in the second posttreatment decade. Cancer Med. 2017;6(7):1827–36. https://doi.org/10.1002/cam4.1103. Epub 31 May 2017.
17. Sanda MG, Dunn RL, Michalski J, Sandler HM, Northouse L, Hembroff L, Lin X, Greenfield TK, Litwin MS, Saigal CS, Mahadevan A, Klein E, Kibel A, Pisters LL, Kuban D, Kaplan I, Wood D, Ciezki J, Shah N, Wei JT. Quality of life and satisfaction with outcome among prostate-cancer survivors. N Engl J Med. 2008;358(12):1250–61. https://doi.org/10.1056/NEJMoa074311.
18. Goonewardene SS, Gillatt D, Persad R. A systematic review of PFE pre-prostatectomy. J Robot Surg. 2018;12:1–4.

19. Siegel AL. Pelvic floor muscle training in males: practical applications. Urology. 2014;84(1):1–7. https://doi.org/10.1016/j.urol-
ogy.2014.03.016. Epub 10 May 2014.
20. Nagpal AS, Moody EL. Interventional management for pelvic
pain. Phys Med Rehabil Clin N Am. 2017;28(3):621–46. https://
doi.org/10.1016/j.pmr.2017.03.011. Epub 27 May 2017.
21. Plancarte R, Amescua C, Patt RB, Aldrete JA. Superior hypogastric plexus block for pelvic cancer pain. Anesthesiology.
1990;73(2):236–9.
22. Ahmed DG, Mohamed MF, Mohamed SA. Superior hypogastric plexus combined with ganglion impar neurolytic blocks
for pelvic and/or perineal cancer pain relief. Pain Physician.
2015;18(1):E49–56.
23. American Cancer Society. Cancer facts and figures 2018. Atlanta:
American Cancer Society; 2018.
24. Hammer SM, Brown JC, Segal S, Chu CS, Schmitz KH. Cancer-
related impairments influence physical activity in uterine cancer
survivors. Med Sci Sports Exerc. 2014;46(12):2195.
25. Biglia N, Zanfagnin V, Daniele A, Robba E, Bounous VE. Lower
body lymphedema in patients with gynecologic cancer.
Anticancer Res. 2017;37(8):4005–15.
26. Ryan M, Stainton MC, Jaconelli C, Watts S, MacKenzie P,
Mansberg T. The experience of lower limb lymphedema for
women after treatment for gynecologic cancer. Oncol Nurs
Forum. 2003;30(3):417–23.
27. Beesley VL, Rowlands IJ, Hayes SC, Janda M, O'Rourke P,
Marquart L, Quinn MA, Spurdle AB, Obermair A, Brand A,
Oehler MK. Incidence, risk factors and estimates of a woman's
risk of developing secondary lower limb lymphedema and
lymphedema-specific supportive care needs in women treated
for endometrial cancer. Gynecol Oncol. 2015;136(1):87–93.
28. Executive Committee. Lymphology. 2016;49(4):170–84.
29. Bakar Y, Tuğral A. Lower extremity lymphedema management
after gynecologic cancer surgery: a review of current management strategies. Ann Vasc Surg. 2017;44:442–50. https://doi.
org/10.1016/j.avsg.2017.03.197. Epub 5 May 2017.
30. Do JH, Choi KH, Ahn JS, Jeon JY. Effects of a complex rehabilitation program on edema status, physical function, and quality
of life in lower-limb lymphedema after gynecological cancer surgery. Gynecol Oncol. 2017;147(2):450–5. https://doi.org/10.1016/j.
ygyno.2017.09.003. Epub 20 Sep 2017.

31. Nieves-Neira W, Kim JJ, Matei D. Hormonal strategies in gyne-
    cologic cancer: bridging biology and therapy. Gynecol Oncol.
    2018;150(2):207–10. https://doi.org/10.1016/j.ygyno.2018.06.005.
    Epub 20 Jun 2018.
32. Ramaseshan AS, Felton J, Roque D, Rao G, Shipper AG, Sanses
    TVD. Pelvic floor disorders in women with gynecologic malig-
    nancies: a systematic review. Int Urogynecol J. 2018;29(4):459–
    76. https://doi.org/10.1007/s00192-017-3467-4. Epub 19 Sep 2017.
33. Arnouk A, De E, Rehfuss A, Cappadocia C, Dickson S, Lian
    F. Physical, complementary, and alternative medicine in the
    treatment of pelvic floor disorders. Curr Urol Rep. 2017;18(6):47.
    https://doi.org/10.1007/s11934-017-0694-7.
34. Yang EJ, Lim JY, Rah UW, Kim YB. Effect of a pelvic floor mus-
    cle training program on gynecologic cancer survivors with pelvic
    floor dysfunction: a randomized controlled trial. Gynecol Oncol.
    2012;125(3):705–11. https://doi.org/10.1016/j.ygyno.2012.03.045.
    Epub 1 Apr 2012.
35. Rutledge TL, Rogers R, Lee SJ, Muller CY. A pilot random-
    ized control trial to evaluate pelvic floor muscle training
    for urinary incontinence among gynecologic cancer survivors.
    Gynecol Oncol. 2014;132(1):154–8. https://doi.org/10.1016/j.
    ygyno.2013.10.024. Epub 29 Oct 2013.
36. Fukushima H, Nakanishi Y, Kataoka M, Tobisu K, Koga
    F. Prognostic significance of sarcopenia in patients with meta-
    static renal cell carcinoma. J Urol. 2016;195(1):26–32. https://doi.
    org/10.1016/j.juro.2015.08.071. Epub 17 Aug 2015.
37. Yip SM, Heng DY, Tang PA. Review of the interaction between
    body composition and clinical outcomes in metastatic renal cell
    cancer treated with targeted therapies. J Kidney Cancer VHL.
    2016;3(1):12–22. https://doi.org/10.15586/jkcvhl.2016.45. eCollec-
    tion 2016.
38. Smith BW, Joseph JR, Saadeh YS, La Marca F, Szerlip NJ,
    Schermerhorn TC, Spratt DE, Younge KC, Park P. Radiosurgery
    for treatment of renal cell metastases to spine: a systematic
    review of the literature. World Neurosurg. 2018;109:e502–9.
    https://doi.org/10.1016/j.wneu.2017.10.011. Epub 13 Oct 2017.

Chapter 6
Rehabilitation of Individuals with Head and Neck Cancers

Alba Azola and R. Samuel Mayer

Case Presentation

A 70-year-old man presents to your office with T1N1 stage III laryngeal cancer. He is a smoker with mild COPD. He is starting chemotherapy and radiotherapy, and is scheduled to have a laryngectomy and radical neck dissection in 3 weeks.

What further information do you need to know in order to plan his rehabilitation? What complications and impairments might you anticipate?

Anatomic Regions

In order to rehabilitate patients with head and neck cancers (HNC), physiatrists should familiarize themselves with the basic anatomy of the region. Cancers of the head and neck encompass lesions at oral cavity, pharynx, larynx, salivary glands, and paranasal sinuses. The location and origin of the

A. Azola · R. S. Mayer (✉)
Department of Physical Medicine and Rehabilitation, Johns Hopkins University School of Medicine, Baltimore, MD, USA
e-mail: aazola1@jhmi.edu; rmayer2@jhmi.edu

© Springer Nature Switzerland AG 2020
J. Baima, A. Khanna (eds.), *Cancer Rehabilitation*,
https://doi.org/10.1007/978-3-030-44462-4_6

Head and Neck Cancer Regions

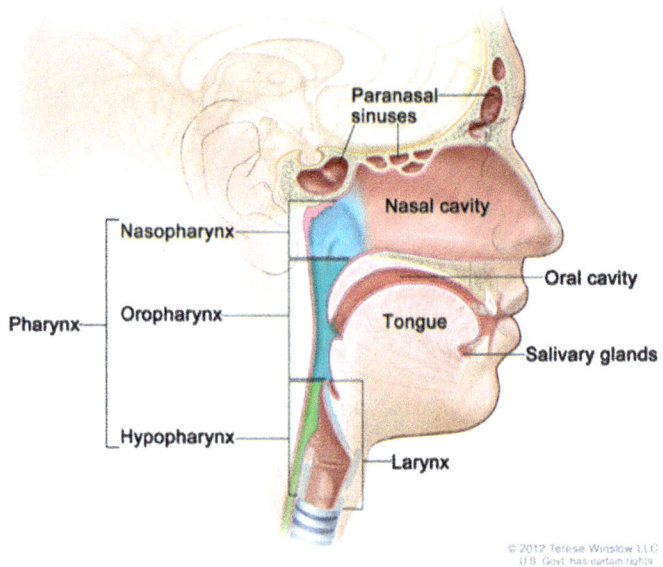

FIGURE 6.1 Picture in cancer rehabilitation. Page 305, Fig. 22.1 [1]

tumors is critical for staging, treatment plan, and management, as well as impairment profile. Figure 6.1 shows a dia-
gram of the main regions in the head and neck (H&N).

Epidemiology and Survival

Cancer of the head and neck represents 5.6% of all cancers in
the United States [2], and it predominantly affects males, with
an M:F ratio of 3:1 [3]. There has been a steady rise in the
incidence of head and neck cancers over the past decade and

this trend will continue in both developed and underdeveloped countries to the year 2030 [4].

The main etiologies in head and neck malignancies are exposure to tobacco products, alcohol consumption, and viral etiologies such as human papilloma virus in oropharyngeal cancer and Epstein-Barr virus in nasopharyngeal cancer.

The vast majority of malignancies involving the lip, oral cavity, and pharynx are squamous cell carcinomas. Approximately 500,000 new cases of head and neck squamous cell carcinoma are reported worldwide every year, and 40,000 of these are diagnosed in the USA [5]. Over the past two decades, there has been a shift in the primary site distribution, with an increase in oropharyngeal cancers and a decrease in tumors located in the larynx and hypopharynx. Parallel with this change of prevalence in primary sites, we have observed a shift on the risk factor profile, with an overall decrease in smoking and the identification of high-risk oncogenic human papilloma virus as a risk factor for oropharyngeal tumors.

The HPV positive oropharyngeal cancer patients tend to be middle age (<60 years old), non-smoking, Caucasian males of higher socioeconomic status with a history of multiple sexual partners. The prognosis for the HPV positive patient is substantially better, with a 2-year overall survival of 94% versus 58% in the HPV negative tobacco related cancers [6]. This has driven major changes in the 2017 head and neck cancer staging manual, including distinct staging systems for HPV+ (p16+) and HPV- tumors with corresponding improved prediction of survival; incorporation of depth of invasion of oral cavity lesions to the T designation; and addition of extra nodal extension to the N pathologic criteria [6]. See Tables 6.1 and 6.2.

The 5-year Cumulative Index Function (CIF) of cancer-specific mortality of squamous cell carcinomas of head and neck is 26.7%, while the competing mortality (deaths from other causes) adds another 12.7%; hence overall survival is 60.6% [7].

TABLE 6.1 Anatomic stage and prognostic groups for human papilloma virus-associated (p-16 positive) oropharyngeal cancer

T Category	N Category			
	N0	**N1**	**N2**	**N3**
T0	NA	I	II	III
T1	I	I	II	III
T2	I	I	II	III
T3	II	II	II	III
T4	III	III	III	III

[a]Any evidence of metastasis is Stage VI
Adapted from Deschler DG, Moore MG, Smith RV, eds. Quick Reference Guide to TNM Staging of Head and Neck Cancer and Neck Dissection Classification, 4th ed. Alexandria, VA: American Academy of Otolaryngology–Head and Neck Surgery Foundation, 2014

TABLE 6.2 Anatomic stage and prognostic groups for nonhuman papilloma virus-associated (p-16 negative) oropharyngeal cancer

T Category	N Category			
	N0	**N1**	**N2**[a,b,c]	**N3**
T1	I	III	IVA	IVB
T2	II	III	IVA	IVB
T3	III	III	IVA	IVB
T4a	IVA	IVA	IVA	IVB
T4b	IVB	IVB	IVB	IVB

[a]Any evidence of metastasis is Stage VIC
Adapted from Deschler DG, Moore MG, Smith RV, eds. Quick Reference Guide to TNM Staging of Head and Neck Cancer and Neck Dissection Classification, 4th ed. Alexandria, VA: American Academy of Otolaryngology–Head and Neck Surgery Foundation, 2014

Location-Specific Functional Impairments

The result of these epidemiologic changes in the head and neck cancer population is a growing number of younger survivors at risk of significant impairments associated with the disease process itself and treatment toxicities, highlighting the importance of functional preservation. The loss, or reduction, of function associated with head and neck malignancies and its treatment toxicities have a profound impact on the survivor's quality of life. A multicenter international study looking at functional outcomes in H&N cancer patients revealed that the most common patient-reported impairments are disfigurement (82%), dysphagia (75%), and changes in articulation (67%). These restrict basic functions, such as the ability to ingest food and communicate with others, as well as participate in leisurely and community activities [5]. Other common reported complaints affecting quality of life include dysphonia, trismus, xerostomia, dental cavities, tracheostomy tube dependence, neck and shoulder dysfunction, neuropathy, and lymphedema.

Impairments can be categorized by the etiology of the deficits including those caused by the primary tumor, metastatic disease, and acute and chronic treatment side effects. The deficits associated with the primary tumor will depend on its anatomical location, size, and degree of loco-regional spread. Impairments commonly involve oral and/oropharyngeal dysphagia, changes in articulation, resonance, phonation, localized and referred pain, vocal cord dysfunction, and hearing loss. See Table 6.3.

TABLE 6.3 Primary tumor location specific consideration and impairments in head and neck cancer

Location	Site-specific consideration	Functional impairment
Lips, oral cavity, oral tongue	Early diagnosis due to visibility (i.e., routine dental evaluation) Sensory impairments can further limit functional recovery Dental rehabilitation Osteoradionecrosis after Radiation to the mandible	Oral swallow (bolus preparation and oral control of bolus) Speech (articulation) Xerostomia secondary to radiation to salivary glands

(continued)

TABLE 6.3 (continued)

Location	Site-specific consideration	Functional impairment
Oropharynx and base of tongue	Trismus secondary to pterygoid involvement or fibrosis Velopharyngeal insufficiency from involvement of soft palate Fibrosis to upper esophageal sphincter from radiation treatment Pain (referred to ear and neck)	Oral and pharyngeal swallow (bolus propulsion, poor pharyngeal contraction, UES dysfunction) Trismus (decreased range of motion of jaw) Speech (articulation, hypo/ hypernasal speech) Xerostomia secondary to radiation to salivary glands
Nasopharynx	Mainstay of treatment is radiation, with wide field, including brain Lhermitte syndrome can be seen post radiation Osteoradionecrosis of skull base Bulbar palsy as late effect of radiation	Nasal regurgitation (velopharyngeal insufficiency) Hyponasal speech Neurocognitive deficits Hearing loss (eustachian tube involvement)
Laryngeal	Total laryngectomy associated with good swallowing outcome and serviceable voice (electrolarynx or tracheoesophageal prosthesis) Radiation associated with laryngeal edema and fibrosis as well as restricted laryngeal movement	Pharyngeal dysphagia (airway protection compromised with high risk of aspiration) Hypophonia/ dysphonia Vocal cord dysfunction, glottic compromise

TABLE 6.3 (continued)

Location	Site-specific consideration	Functional impairment
Hypopharyngeal	Higher risk of metastasis Strictures with stenosis of upper esophagus	Pharyngeal dysphagia (outlet obstruction, poor pharyngeal contraction) Vocal cord dysfunction

The presence of loco-regional spread to cervical lymph nodes has a strong negative effect on prognosis and increased disease recurrence in the head and neck cancer patient. Furthermore, finding extracapsular spread (ECS) in the involved lymph nodes decreases the 5-year survival from 70% to 27% [8]. ECS is a biological marker of aggressive disease and one of the most important prognostic markers, leading to consideration of aggressive multimodal treatment in its presence.

Treatment-Specific Functional Impairments

Treatment of head and neck cancer varies by tumor histology, location, and staging. However, most of the regimens involve combinations of chemotherapy, radiation therapy, and surgery. Many of the protocols involve giving chemotherapy and/or radiation prior to surgical resection, unlike protocols for most other cancers, where chemotherapy or radiotherapy occur after resection.

Chemotherapy Side Effects

The most common chemotherapeutic regimen for squamous cell head and neck cancer is a combination of cisplatin and fluorouracil. Cisplatin can cause fatigue, peripheral neuropathy, myalgia, vision changes, and gout, as well as alopecia, renal impairment, and myelosuppression. In rare cases, strokes and reversible posterior leukoencephalopathy have been reported.

Fluorouracil also causes fatigue, myelosuppression, and alopecia, but also causes a lot of acute gastrointestinal side effects (nausea, vomiting, diarrhea, and mucositis), and more rarely cardiotoxicity and cerebellar ataxia. Taxanes are also used with some frequency, and can cause peripheral neuropathy as well as arthralgia and myalgia. Pembrolizumab is a newer immunotherapy agent being used off-label for head and neck cancers. It also can cause fatigue, musculoskeletal pain, and in rare cases peripheral neuropathy. It has the potential to cause immune-mediated syndromes, including Stevens-Johnson syndrome and myasthenia gravis.

Radiation Therapy

Radiation fibrosis can occur in the field of treatment. It can manifest as pulmonary fibrosis when the lungs are involved, but also cause fibrosis of skin, soft tissue, and muscle. This can lead to torticollis and trismus, and cause significant pain. Abnormal jaw, neck, and shoulder motion

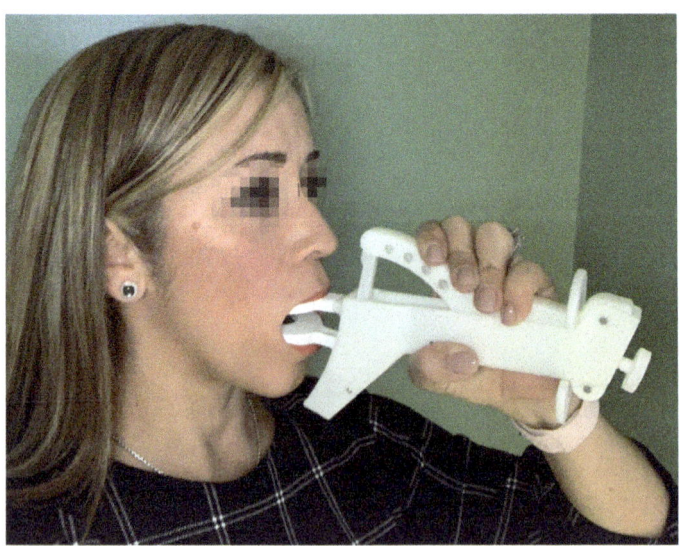

Figure 6.2 Jaw Dynasplint – PC Dr. Alba Azola

can result. Treatment of this can include range of motion exercise, taping, bracing (Fig. 6.2). Pentoxifylline with vitamin E has shown some promise in reducing symptoms [9]. In some cases, treatment with botulinum toxin injections may help [10].

Dysphagia occurs in approximately 75% of HNC patients, and is especially associated with radiation therapy (although local tumor burden and surgical resection also influence this). It can occur early in the course of the disease or can be late in onset. A recent study [11] demonstrated that prophylactic treatment with gabapentin during radiotherapy significantly decreased the subsequent incidence and severity of dysphagia.

Surgery

Surgical resections can result in significant impairments depending on the location and extent of the operation. Nasopharyngeal resections can be quite disfiguring, with resultant emotional distress in many cases. Glossectomy for tongue cancers may result in significant oral phase dysphagia if anterior, and oropharyngeal dysphagia if posterior. It also, of course, causes dysarthria. Laryngectomy is disfiguring, and causes aphonia or dysphonia. This can be mitigated with electrolarynx devices or with tracheo-esophageal prostheses. The latter requires surgical creation of a tracheo-esophageal fistula and placement of a one-way valve that allows air to move into the esophagus allowing the patient, with proper training, to produce speech. In cases where lymph node metastasis occurs, a radical or modified radical neck dissection may be indicated. This can involve resection of the sternocleidomastoid, with resultant limitation in range of motion. The recurrent laryngeal nerve may be damaged or sacrificed, with resultant severe dysphagia and dysphonia. The spinal accessory nerve also lies in close proximity, and injury of it will lead to inferolateral winging of the scapula due to trapezius weakness. This results in shoulder pain, weakness, and limited range of motion. Early intervention with physical therapy as well as electrical stimulation and taping of the scapula has been showed to improve shoulder functional outcomes [12].

Social Participation Restrictions

Taylor et al. [13] identified treatment with chemotherapy, neck dissection, and pain score as factors that increased the odds of disability, and estimated that 52% of patients working before diagnosis were able to return to work. A second study looking at return to work for H&N cancer patients younger than 65 years-old found that 71% of those working prior to diagnosis retuned to work within 6 months of end of treatment, emphasizing age and level of education as favorable factors [14].

Case Presentation Continued…
Our patient underwent "prehab" prior to his surgery with speech and physical therapy; he also took gabapentin during his radiation treatments. Unfortunately, he had involvement of his recurrent laryngeal and spinal accessory nerves and has dysphagia as well as scapular winging and limited neck range of motion. He continues to work with PT and SLP. He has an electro-larynx, and is considering a TE prosthesis. Due to his social anxiety with his appearance, you have referred him to psychology. He is very grateful for the rehab team's efforts.

Multiple Choice Questions

1. What percent of cancers does cancer of the head and neck represent?

    A. 1–5%
    B. 5–10%
    C. 10–15%
    D. 15–20%
    E. 20–25%

2. Which of the following is/are risk factor(s) for head and neck cancer?

    A. Tobacco use
    B. Epstein Barr virus
    C. Human papilloma virus
    D. Alcohol use
    E. All of the above

3. What is the significance of extracapsular spread in head and neck cancer?

   A. Symptoms of hearing loss more likely
   B. Increases the 5-year survival
   C. Biologic marker of aggressive disease
   D. Does not affect prognosis

4. Which chemotherapy agent used in head and neck cancer causes fatigue, peripheral neuropathy, myalgia, vision changes, and gout?

   A. Fluorouracil
   B. Cisplatin
   C. Pembrolizumab
   D. Pentoxifylline

5. What supportive devices are available post-laryngectomy?

   A. Electrolarynx
   B. Scrambler therapy
   C. Tracheo-esophageal prosthetic
   D. A and C

Answers

1. B
2. E
3. C
4. B
5. D

References

1. Stubblefield MD. Cancer rehabilitation 2E: principles and practice. New York: Springer Publishing Company; 2018.
2. Siegel RL, Miller KD, Jemal A. Cancer statistics, 2019. CACancer J Clin. 2019;69(1):7–34.
3. Stoyanov GS, Kitanova M, Dzhenkov DL, Ghenev P, Sapundzhiev N. Demographics of head and neck cancer patients: a single institution experience. Cureus. 2017;9(7):e1418.

 4. Gupta B, Johnson NW, Kumar N. Global epidemiology of head and neck cancers: a continuing challenge. Oncology. 2016;91(1):13–23.
 5. Gillison ML, Chaturvedi AK, Anderson WF, Fakhry C. Epidemiology of human papillomavirus–positive head and neck squamous cell carcinoma. J Clin Oncol. 2015;33(29):3235.
 6. Lydiatt WM, Patel SG, O'Sullivan B, et al. Head and neck cancers—major changes in the American Joint Committee on Cancer eighth edition cancer staging manual. CA Cancer J Clin. 2017;67(2):122–37.
 7. Shen W, Sakamoto N, Yang L. Model to predict cause-specific mortality in patients with head and neck adenoid cystic carcinoma: a competing risk analysis. Ann Surg Oncol. 2017;24(8):2129–36.
 8. Chai RL, Rath TJ, Johnson JT, et al. Accuracy of computed tomography in the prediction of extracapsular spread of lymph node metastases in squamous cell carcinoma of the head and neck. JAMA Otolaryngol Head Neck Surg. 2013;139(11):1187–94.
 9. Kaidar-Person O, Marks LB, Jones EL. Pentoxifylline and vitamin E for treatment or prevention of radiation-induced fibrosis in patients with breast cancer. Breast J. 2018;24(5):816–9.
10. Stubblefield MD, Levine A, Custodio CM, Fitzpatrick T. The role of botulinum toxin type A in the radiation fibrosis syndrome: a preliminary report. Arch Phys Med Rehabil. 2008;89(3):417–21.
11. Bar Ad V, Weinstein G, Dutta PR, et al. Gabapentin for the treatment of pain syndrome related to radiation-induced mucositis in patients with head and neck cancer treated with concurrent chemoradiotherapy. Cancer. 2010;116(17):4206–13.
12. McGarvey AC, Hoffman GR, Osmotherly PG, Chiarelli PE. Maximizing shoulder function after accessory nerve injury and neck dissection surgery: a multicenter randomized controlled trial. Head Neck. 2015;37(7):1022–31.
13. Taylor JC, Terrell JE, Ronis DL, et al. Disability in patients with head and neck cancer. Arch Otolaryngol Head Neck Surg. 2004;130(6):764–9.
14. Verdonck-de Leeuw IM, van Bleek W, Leemans CR, de Bree R. Employment and return to work in head and neck cancer survivors. Oral Oncol. 2010;46(1):56–60.

Chapter 7
Cancer of the Lymphoid, Hematopoietic, and Related Tissue

Diana Molinares, Sara Parke, and Ekta Gupta

Introduction

Cancers of the lymphoid, hematopoietic, and related tissues are also known as blood cancers. Blood cancers are often characterized by the uncontrolled proliferation of abnormal blood cells, which reduces the production of normal blood cells and impairs blood function [1]. Blood has many important functions including transporting oxygen to the vital organs, carrying waste products to the liver and kidneys for disposal, forming clots, fighting infection, and regulating body temperature. According to the American Society of Hematology, blood cancers can be classified into three types: leukemia, lymphoma, and myeloma [2] (Table 7.1).

Blood is a body fluid that is primarily made up of two components, plasma (55%) and blood cells (45%) [2]. Blood stem cells differentiate into either myeloid or lymphoid stem cells as depicted in Fig. 7.1, and then into committed progenitors.

The authors Diana Molinares and Sara Parke are co-first authors.

D. Molinares · S. Parke · E. Gupta (✉)
Department of Palliative, Rehabilitation and Integrative Medicine,
University of Texas MD Anderson Cancer Center,
Houston, TX, USA
e-mail: egupta@mdanderson.org

© Springer Nature Switzerland AG 2020
J. Baima, A. Khanna (eds.), *Cancer Rehabilitation*,
https://doi.org/10.1007/978-3-030-44462-4_7

TABLE 7.1 Classification of hematological neoplasms (simplified from WHO 2017 classification) [6]

Myeloid neoplasms	Acute myeloid leukemia (AML)
From myeloid progenitors	Myeloproliferative neoplasms (MPN) *(Chronic myeloid leukemia, Polycythemia vera, Essential thrombocythemia, Primary myelofibrosis, Others)*
	Myelodysplastic syndrome (MDS)
	Myelodysplastic/myeloproliferative neoplasms
Lymphoid neoplasms	Acute lymphoblastic leukemia/lymphoma (ALL)
From mature B- or T-cells or lymphoid progenitors	Chronic lymphocytic leukemia (CLL)
	B-cell non-Hodgkin lymphoma (NHL) *Diffuse large B-cell lymphoma, follicular lymphoma, mantle cell lymphoma, marginal zone lymphoma, lymphoplasmacytic lymphoma*
	Hodgkin lymphoma (HL)
	Mature T- and NK-cell neoplasms *Peripheral T-cell lymphoma, anaplastic large cell lymphoma, adult T-cell leukemia/lymphoma, mycosis fungoides/Sézary syndrome, primary cutaneous peripheral T-cell lymphomas, others*
Histiocytic and dendritic cell neoplasms	Histiocytic sarcoma, Langerhans cell histiocytosis, Erdheim-Chest disease, others
From dendritic cells or histiocytes	Blastic plasmacytoid dendritic cell neoplasm (BPDCN)
Others	Mastocytosis

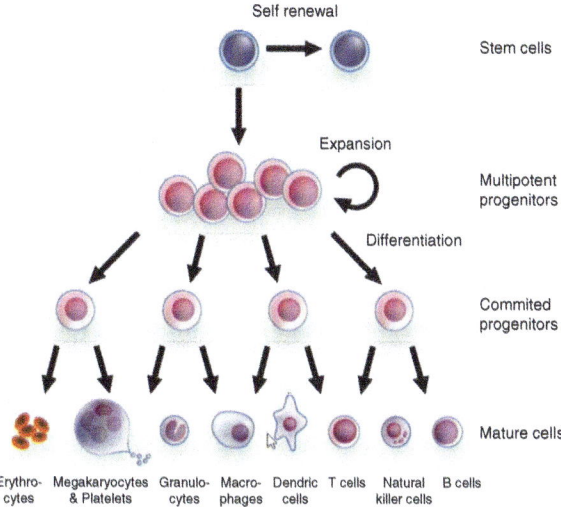

FIGURE 7.1 This figure depicts the hematopoietic stem cell tree, with differentiation into each mature cell as discussed above [4]

Myeloid stem cells differentiate into red blood cells, platelets, and myeloblasts which produce granulocytes (eosinophils, basophils, and neutrophils). Lymphoid stems cells differentiate into lymphoblasts, which then produce B lymphocytes (B-cells), T lymphocytes (T-cells), and natural killer cells (NK-cells). White blood cells are granulocytes, NK-cells, T-Cells, and B-cells [3]. When infection is present, B-cells transform into plasma cells, which produce antibodies [3].

Leukemia

Leukemia results from an abnormal proliferation of blood cells. Depending on which cell line the abnormal cell originates from, the leukemia is named (i.e., Myeloid = acute myeloid leukemia, B or T cell = acute lymphoblastic leukemia). In Western countries, chronic lymphocytic leukemia (CLL) is the most frequently seen leukemia and is approximately 30% of all leukemias in the United States. Meanwhile, acute lymphoblastic leukemia (ALL) is the most common malignancy in children and it is very uncommon in adults [5]. Patients can present with the effects of the decreased count of normal blood cell lines (leukopenia, anemia, and thrombocytopenia) as they are being replaced by leukemic blast forms. The goal of the oncological treatment is to decrease the counts of blast cells in the peripheral blood and bone marrow.

Lymphomas

Lymphomas are lymphoproliferative disorders derived from the lymphoid stem cell. Also identified by their cell lineage, mature B-Cell, T-cell, and Natural Killer-cell neoplasms can be of several types [6]. There are some with no strict normal cellular counterpart, such as hairy cell leukemia, and others with genetic aberrations [6]. Clinical features often include painless, swollen lymph nodes, mediastinal mass, fever, night sweats, pruritus, weight loss, and fatigue.

Myeloma

Myeloma is a proliferative disorder of plasma cells [7]. Similar to plasma cells, myeloma cells make antibody-like proteins called monoclonal proteins or M-proteins [3]. Unlike antibodies, however, M-proteins are produced in an uncontrolled fashion and do not effectively target infectious agents. Myeloma cells are produced in the bone marrow and travel through the blood stream where they collect at multiple sites [8]. Uncontrolled proliferation of myeloma cells has many deleterious effects, including: reduced production of normal antibodies, which increases the body's vulnerability to infection; increased production of abnormal antibodies, which leads to hyperviscosity and organ damage, particularly renal dysfunction; and increased bone destruction, which causes pain and fractures [8]. Commonly ordered laboratory tests include serum free light-chain assay, serum protein electrophoresis (SPEP) and urine protein electrophoresis (UPEP), bone marrow aspirate, and biopsy, and commonly ordered imaging includes whole body MRI, CT without contrast, or PET/CT [3]. See Table 7.2 for details.

TABLE 7.2 Classification and diagnostic criteria of plasma cell neoplasms [7, 9, 10]

MGUS	Presence of a monoclonal protein at a concentration <30 g/L Bone marrow with <10% monoclonal plasma cells Absence of myeloma-defining events (see below)
Smoldering myeloma (asymptomatic)	Serum monoclonal protein ≥30 g/L or urinary monoclonal protein ≥500 mg/24 h and/or clonal bone marrow plasma cells 10–59% Absence of myeloma-defining events (see below) or amyloidosis
Multiple myeloma (symptomatic)	Myeloma cells ≥10% or biopsy-proven bony or extramedullary plasmacytoma and ≥1 myeloma-defining criteria: I. Evidence of end organ damage (CRAB) II. Any one of the following biomarkers: clonal bone marrow plasma cell percentage ≥60%, >1 focal lesions on MRI, involved-to-uninvolved serum free light-chain ratio ≥100
Solitary plasmacytoma	Biopsy-proven solitary lesion of bone or soft tissue with evidence of clonal plasma cells Normal bone marrow with no evidence of clonal plasma cells Absence of myeloma-defining events (see above)
POEMS syndrome	Paraneoplastic condition characterized by polyneuropathy, organomegaly, endocrinopathy, monoclonal gammopathy, and skin changes
Systemic AL amyloidosis	Presence of amyloid-related organ damage (e.g., renal, liver, heart, gastrointestinal tract, peripheral nerves) Positive amyloid staining by Congo red in any tissue Evidence of amyloid light-chain deposits by mass spectrometry or immunoelectron microscopy Evidence of monoclonal plasma cell disorder

MGUS monoclonal gammopathy of undetermined significance, *CRAB* Hypercalcemia, Renal insufficiency, Anemia, osteolytic Bone lesions

Exercise in Hematopoietic Cell Transplant Patients

Although more research is needed to determine the intensity and type of exercise recommended in patients with hematopoietic cancer-related fatigue, exercise is believed to improve fatigue, mood, sleep and functional capacity [16–18]. Some of the benefits of exercise on the treatment of cancer-related fatigue are believed to be secondary to decreased inflammation [16, 19]. Exercise is especially important for patients undergoing hematopoietic cell transplant as a minimum functional level is required to undergo a transplant. See Table 7.3 for details. In these cases, exercise to combat the effects of cancer or its treatment may be considered prehabilitation for transplant surgery. (See Chap. 1 for the definition of prehabilitation.)

Clinical Case

An 81-year-old man presents with the history of monoclonal gammopathy of undetermined significance (MGUS), initially diagnosed at age 66. He remained under observation for 2 years before his disease progressed to multiple myeloma (MM). He then underwent radiation to the skull and femur followed by a course of chemotherapy with thalidomide and dexamethasone. He also underwent an autologous stem cell transplant without lasting functional impairment. At age 71, thalidomide was discontinued due to development of progressive length-dependent polyneuropathy. He had numbness and reduced proprioception in the feet that required him to use a walker. Nonetheless, he continued to work full-time at a job that required frequent airplane travel. At age 80, he returned with sudden-onset bilateral leg weakness and incontinence. He was found to have a biopsy-confirmed plasma cell neoplasm at T9 with resulting Bilsky grade 3 cord compression. He was also found to have a pulmonary embolism requiring therapeutic anticoagulation. He was not a surgical

TABLE 7-3 Impairments and therapy prescription considerations [5, 11–15]

	Impairments	Therapy prescription considerations
Diagnosis	Fatigue Thrombocytopenia Bruising or bleeding Frequent infections Renal dysfunction Bone pain and fractures (vertebral bodies, ribs, skull, shoulder, hip) [3] Anemia Lymphedema Cachexia Hyperleukocytosis (WBC or leukoblast count>100,000/μL)	*Thrombocytopenia* >20,000 platelets/μL: No restrictions 10,000–20,000/μL: No resistive exercise. Fall precautions 5000–9999/μL: No resistive exercises and bed/chair exercise <5000/μL: Discuss with oncology team or consider deferring treatment [11] *Anemia* <8 g/dL (severe anemia): Close monitoring of symptoms and vital signs with intervention [5, 12] Adjust rehabilitation plan based on risk of pathologic fracture (Mirels' criteria and spinal instability neoplastic score (SINS)) [12]
Treatment	**Radiation therapy** *For focal bone pain due to pathological fracture, or solitary plasmacytoma, or directed to specific lymphoma* Local skin reaction Local hair loss Fatigue Nausea Diarrhea Fibrosis of local tissue with potential decrease range of motion (ROM)	Fatigue and anemia reduce exercise tolerance Protect areas of skin breakdown to prevent breakdown Monitor cardiopulmonary function patient with prior radiation to the thorax [13]

(continued)

TABLE 7.3 (continued)

	Impairments	Therapy prescription considerations
	Surgery *To repair fractures or remove a solitary plasmacytoma*	Impairments depend on procedure Weight-bearing restrictions Edema Deconditioning/weakness Sensory-changes Scarring Pain	Procedure dependent Early mobilization is encouraged [12] Plan of care with activity restrictions that facilitates tissue healing
	Chemotherapy/targeted therapy *Used as first line for most patients. There are many different potential agents including targeted therapy immunomodulators, monoclonal antibodies to control systemic disease*	Impairments depend on type of therapy Nausea Diarrhea or constipation Bruising and bleeding Fevers and infections Blood clot Neuropathy Rash Myalgia Alopecia Mouth sores Cachexia	Agent dependent Awareness of potential side effects of medication in use Awareness of the nadir of blood cell counts due to chemotherapy effect (see neutropenia below) Barrier precautions in immunocompromised patients Awareness to differentiate between therapy-induced gastrointestinal effects and infection Importance of nutrition Energy conservation exercises

Steroids *Can be used alone, or in combination with chemotherapy/targeted therapy to treat inflammation*	Increased appetite Weight gain Insomnia Edema Dyspepsia Irritability Psychosis Increased risk of infection Delayed wound healing Fracture Myopathy (proximal)	Weight bearing exercises may prevent frail bones and fractures [14] Fall education and safety to avoid fractures Glucose control Gastrointestinal prophylaxis for ulcers See myopathy below
Stem cell transplant *Autologous or allogeneic; used in patients with active hematological cancer who have been treated systemically and either had a complete response or no response*	Fatigue Infection Bleeding Mouth sores Deconditioning Critical illness myopathy/polyneuropathy Graft versus host disease (skin, intestines, muscles, joints, eyes, or liver)	***Immunosuppression*** **>11,000 cells/μL or <4000 cells/μL:** Symptom-based approach, monitor for fever **<1500 neutrophils/μL (neutropenia):** Neutropenic precautions based on facility guidelines Neutropenia is not a contraindication to rehabilitation [12] Antibiotic, antifungal, and antiviral prophylaxis for immunocompromised patients Immunosuppressed patients to avoid public gyms and pools [5], no fresh fruits or vegetables See thrombocytopenia and anemia above

(continued)

TABLE 7.3 (continued)

	Impairments	Therapy prescription considerations
Survivorship	GVHD requiring immunosuppression or steroids can result in: Weight-bearing or range-of-motion restriction Malnutrition Weakness Sarcopenia Asthenia Vision change Neuropathy Decreased proprioception and balance Increased risk of falls	***Sclerodermatous contractures*** Contracture preventions: ROM exercises – splinting ***Myopathy*** Fall prevention and strengthening focused on proximal muscles Bracing for weak muscles. Adaptive equipment ***Peripheral neuropathy*** Bracing for motor weakness Wound prevention Medication management ***Deconditioning*** Exercise program [15] Nutrition referral focused on ensuring protein intake

candidate and underwent intensity-modulated radiation therapy (IMRT) for 13 fractions. During his radiation treatment, he was transferred to acute inpatient rehabilitation for management of the sequela of spinal cord injury. His rehabilitation admission was interrupted by complications related to fungal pneumonia. He was then discharged from the acute oncology service to a skilled nursing facility until his activity tolerance improved to 3 hours per day.

Two months after his presentation with cord compression, the patient underwent posterior segmental instrumentation and fusion of T8-11 for definitive stabilization of the spine. Four days later, he returned to acute inpatient rehabilitation. At that time, his bowel and bladder function had fully recovered as well as his lower extremity strength with the exception of mild symmetrical, proximal weakness likely secondary to steroid myopathy. He continued to have symptoms of length-dependent polyneuropathy that was stable. He remained on acute inpatient rehabilitation for one week. At the time of discharge, he had progressed to a modified independent level for ambulation with a walker and was independent with ADLs.

Multiple Choice Questions

1. Which sequela of multiple myeloma, represented by the acronym "CRAB", are important to consider when developing a rehabilitation program for this patient population?

    A. Cancer Related fatigue, Anemia, Back pain
    B. Hypercalcemia, Renal failure, Agitation, Back pain
    C. Hypercalcemia, Renal failure, Anemia, Bone lesions
    D. Colonic fissure, Renal failure, Agitation, Bone lesions

2. Lymphoma can present with which of the following?

    A. Painless swollen lymph nodes
    B. Mediastinal mass
    C. Unexplained weight loss
    D. All of the above

3. A lymphoma patient undergoes a stem cell transplant and the therapist asks you what activities are okay to do as his platelets are 12,000 platelets/μL. Your response is:

   A. You can do all exercises as tolerated
   B. You can do all aerobic exercises but no resistance exercises
   C. You can only do bed/chair exercises, no resistance exercises

4. Which of the following treatments is recommended to improve fatigue, mood, sleep, and functional capacity:

   A. Methylphenidate
   B. Trazodone
   C. Exercise
   D. Amantadine

5. Which of the following is not a contraindication for physical or occupational therapy?

   A. Platelets of 40,000/μL
   B. White blood cell count of 2000/μL
   C. Hemoglobin of 6.5 g/dL
   D. Lytic lesions of the hips

Answers

1. C
2. D
3. B
4. C
5. A

References

1. Hematology ASo. Blood cancers 2019. Available from: http://www.hematology.org/Patients/Cancers/.
2. Hematology ASo. Blood basics 2019. Available from: http://www.hematology.org/Patients/Basics/.

3. National Comprehensive Cancer Network. Multiple myeloma. Fort Washington: National Comprehensive Cancer Network; 2017.
4. Kursad Turksen PD, editor. Hematopoietic stem cell biology. New York: Humana Press; 2010.
5. Stubblefield MD. Cancer rehabilitation 2E: principles and practice. New York: Springer Publishing Company; 2018.
6. Jaffe ES. Diagnosis and classification of lymphoma: impact of technical advances. Semin Hematol. 2019;56(1):30–6.
7. Rajkumar SV, Dimopoulos MA, Palumbo A, Blade J, Merlini G, Mateos MV, et al. International Myeloma Working Group updated criteria for the diagnosis of multiple myeloma. Lancet Oncol. 2014;15(12):e538–48.
8. Hematology ASo. Myeloma: American Society of Hematology. 2019. Available from: http://www.hematology.org/Patients/Cancers/Myeloma.aspx.
9. Dispenzieri A. POEMS syndrome: 2011 update on diagnosis, risk-stratification, and management. Am J Hematol. 2011;86(7):591–601.
10. Fernandez de Larrea C, Verga L, Morbini P, Klersy C, Lavatelli F, Foli A, et al. A practical approach to the diagnosis of systemic amyloidoses. Blood. 2015;125(14):2239–44.
11. Fu JB, Tennison JM, Rutzen-Lopez IM, Silver JK, Morishita S, Dibaj SS, et al. Bleeding frequency and characteristics among hematologic malignancy inpatient rehabilitation patients with severe thrombocytopenia. Support Care Cancer. 2018;26(9):3135–41.
12. Sebio Garcia R, Yanez Brage MI, Gimenez Moolhuyzen E, Granger CL, Denehy L. Functional and postoperative outcomes after preoperative exercise training in patients with lung cancer: a systematic review and meta-analysis. Interact Cardiovasc Thorac Surg. 2016;23(3):486–97.
13. Bovelli D, Plataniotis G, Roila F, ESMO Guidelines Working Group. Cardiotoxicity of chemotherapeutic agents and radiotherapy-related heart disease: ESMO Clinical Practice Guidelines. Ann Oncol. 2010;21(Suppl 5):v277–82.
14. Daly RM. Exercise and nutritional approaches to prevent frail bones, falls and fractures: an update. Climacteric. 2017;20(2):119–24.
15. Smith SR, Haig AJ, Couriel DR. Musculoskeletal, neurologic, and cardiopulmonary aspects of physical rehabilitation in patients with chronic graft-versus-host disease. Biol Blood Marrow Transplant. 2015;21(5):799–808.

16. Steinberg A, Asher A, Bailey C, Fu JB. The role of physical rehabilitation in stem cell transplantation patients. Support Care Cancer. 2015;23(8):2447–60.
17. Wiskemann J, Huber G. Physical exercise as adjuvant therapy for patients undergoing hematopoietic stem cell transplantation. Bone Marrow Transplant. 2008;41(4):321–9.
18. Baumann FT, Kraut L, Schule K, Bloch W, Fauser AA. A controlled randomized study examining the effects of exercise therapy on patients undergoing haematopoietic stem cell transplantation. Bone Marrow Transplant. 2010;45(2):355–62.
19. Gleeson M, Bishop NC, Stensel DJ, Lindley MR, Mastana SS, Nimmo MA. The anti-inflammatory effects of exercise: mechanisms and implications for the prevention and treatment of disease. Nat Rev Immunol. 2011;11(9):607–15.

Chapter 8
Cancer of the Bone and Connective Tissue

Mathew J. Most and John Haskoor

Introduction

Musculoskeletal tumors may have the greatest potential to affect function. The treatment of orthopedic tumors often requires surgical procedures that significantly alter the limbs. Frequently, a multidisciplinary approach with intense rehabilitation is required in this population.

Principles of Evaluation and Treatment

Histologic diagnosis generally determines treatment options for bone and soft tissue tumors. The goal of musculoskeletal biopsy is to obtain an adequate specimen for diagnosis while keeping contamination to a minimum. Percutaneous methods

M. J. Most (✉)
Division of Orthopedic Oncology, Department of Orthopedics and Physical Rehabilitation, UMass Memorial HealthCare, Worcester, MA, USA
e-mail: mostm@ummhc.org

J. Haskoor
Department of Orthopedics and Physical Rehabilitation, University of Massachusetts Medical School, Worcester, MA, USA
e-mail: john.haskoor@umassmemorial.org

© Springer Nature Switzerland AG 2020   111
J. Baima, A. Khanna (eds.), *Cancer Rehabilitation*,
https://doi.org/10.1007/978-3-030-44462-4_8

exist, such as fine needle aspiration and core biopsy. Core biopsy provides the advantage of obtaining a representative section of tumor where cellular architecture can be evaluated. Lesional tissue can also be obtained as an incisional biopsy (limited incision to access tumor) or excisional biopsy (larger incision with goal to remove grossly visible mass).

It is recommended that the biopsy incision be placed in the area of planned definitive resection. The compartmentalized nature of the appendicular musculoskeletal system provides the advantage of having separated groups of muscles that are invested with thick fascia to eliminate contamination of surrounding tissue and neurovascular structures. Any biopsy tract or associated hematoma is considered contaminated with tumor cells. Therefore, biopsies should always be performed through the compartment that has the tumor to avoid contamination of surrounding tissue.

Definitive resection of the tumor can be described in four main ways, as originally described by Enneking [1]. Intralesional resection removes a portion of the gross specimen with visible tumor tissue left behind. Marginal resection removes the mass en bloc at the interface between gross tumor and surrounding reactive tissue. Wide resection extends the margin around the gross mass into normal appearing tissue but preserves the compartment. Radical resection removes the lesion with its entire surrounding compartment en bloc. Clearly, the extent of resection will not only have a significant effect on risk of local recurrence of disease, but will impact the patient's recovery and rehabilitation.

Limb Salvage Versus Amputation

The primary goal of musculoskeletal tumor surgery is to obtain an adequate resection with negative margins to reduce the risk of local recurrence and/or distant spread. Secondary goals include preserving patient function and cosmesis. Imaging studies are critical to help plan an appropriate resection, and histologic evaluation must be used to confirm complete removal of tumor.

There are many options for limb salvage in tumors of the long bones. Tumors located in the diaphysis or metaphysis can be resected en bloc and reconstructed with allograft bone, autograft bone, endoprostheses, or combinations of these techniques. Technological improvements in implants have allowed for a variety of modular components that can be used to fill defects in a semi-custom manner and provide a functional joint. Additionally, image guidance, robotic assistance, and patient-specific cutting guides are available to ensure accuracy of resection with reduced destruction of healthy tissue by using preoperative imaging to plan resection.

Contraindications to limb salvage include inability to preserve critical neurovascular structures due to tumor involvement that would otherwise leave a poorly or nonfunctional limb. A relative contraindication to limb salvage is gross contamination of the joint with tumor. Traditionally, in skeletally immature patients, involvement of the physis was seen as a contraindication to limb salvage because of issues with growth arrest. Current treatments that address this problem include expandable growth endoprostheses, which can aid in continued lengthening of a limb after tumor resection.

When metastatic tumors, lymphoma, or multiple myeloma are causing significant pain in regions that involve significant difficultly and morbidity to reconstruct and support, percutaneous cementoplasty may be indicated for pain relief during chemotherapy and radiation. Cementoplasty refers to the percutaneous administration of bone cement to reinforce osteolytic lesions to relieve pain. This procedure is indicated for painful osteolytic masses in weight-bearing regions of the skeleton such as the spine, sacrum, acetabulum, and pelvis [2].

When limb salvage is not likely to yield clear margins or spare function, amputation may be indicated. The goal of

Table 8.1 Energy expenditure above baseline for lower extremity amputees

Amputation level	Energy expenditure above baseline (%)
Long transtibial	10
Syme	15
Short transtibial	40
Bilateral transtibial	40
Transfemoral	65

amputation is to amputate at the most distal level possible while ensuring complete removal of malignant tissue. Table 8.1 shows the increase in energy expenditure associated with different amputation levels compared to baseline [3]. Though most of this data refers to traumatic or vascular amputees, it still provides a valuable reference point.

A variety of prosthetic devices exist. In order to determine the appropriate prosthesis, the Centers for Medicare and Medicaid Services (CMS) developed a scoring system to assess the rehab potential of lower extremity amputee patients. These K levels are determined by the treating physician and determine the types of prostheses that will be reimbursed based on functional ability. Table 8.2 shows descriptions of K levels developed by CMS [4].

Cancer of the Bone, Cartilage, and Soft Tissue

Primary malignant tumors of the bone are relatively rare. When a tumor is identified within the axial or appendicular skeleton in a patient over 40 years of age, it is much more commonly secondary to distant metastasis, lymphoma, or multiple myeloma.

TABLE 8.2 Lower limb prosthesis functional levels (K Levels)

K Level	Description
0	This patient does not have the ability or potential to ambulate or transfer safely with or without assistance and a prosthesis does not enhance their quality of life or mobility.
1	Has the ability or potential to use a prosthesis for transfers or ambulation on level surfaces at fixed cadence. Typical of the limited and unlimited household ambulator.
2	Has the ability or potential for ambulation with the ability to traverse low-level environmental barriers such as curbs, stairs, or uneven surfaces. Typical of the limited community ambulator.
3	Has the ability or potential for ambulation with variable cadence. Typical of the community ambulator who has the ability to traverse most environmental barriers and may have vocational, therapeutic, or exercise activity that demands prosthetic utilization beyond simple locomotion.
4	Has the ability or potential for prosthetic ambulation that exceeds basic ambulation skills, exhibiting high impact, stress, or energy levels. Typical of the prosthetic demands of a child, active adult, or athlete.

Metastatic Bone Tumors

The treatment and prognosis of metastatic tumors of the bone is dependent on the primary source of the tumor. Bone is the fourth most common site of metastatic disease following lymphatics, lungs, and liver [5]. Metastatic lesions of the bone typically present as a gradual aching pain of a long bone associated with weight bearing. Other metabolic abnormalities such as hypercalcemia may be the first sign of bony metastasis. Advanced age is a risk factor. Patients may or may not have a history of an associated primary malignancy, and even in patients with known malignancy biopsy can be warranted to definitively rule out a primary bone tumor [6].

The most common primary solid organ tumors resulting in bone metastasis are breast, lung, thyroid, kidney, prostate, and melanoma. Multiple myeloma is an example of a hematopoietic malignancy that results in diffuse bony metastatic disease. Radiation may be used as primary or adjuvant treatment of bone metastasis. Table 8.3 shows the typical appearance, survival, and radiosensitivity of the common metastatic tumors of bone.

Surgical treatment of metastatic bone lesions is indicated for treatment or prevention of fracture and to maintain mobility in cancer patients. Factors that suggest impending fracture or require surgical intervention in the lower extremity, for example, include >50% cortical destruction, a femoral lesion greater than 2.5 cm in diameter, an avulsion fracture of the lesser trochanter, or persistent pain in the hip area 4 weeks following the completion of radiation therapy [7]. Each case needs to be individually evaluated for potential for pathologic fracture, but scoring systems do exist to help

TABLE 8.3 Characteristics of common bone metastatic tumors

Primary	Typical radiographic appearance	5-year survival w/ distant mets	Radiosensitivity
Breast	Mixed	23.8	+++
Lung	Lytic	3.7	++
Thyroid	Lytic	53.9	++
Kidney	Lytic	11.6	−
Prostate	Blastic	27.8	+++
Melanoma	Lytic	15.1	++

TABLE 8.4 Mirels' Score for prediction of pathologic fracture

Score	Location	Appearance	Size (fraction of bone width)	Pain
1	Upper extremity	Blastic	<1/3	Mild
2	Lower extremity	Mixed	1/3 to 2/3	Moderate
3	Peritrochanteric	Lytic	>2/3	Functional

[a]Surgical treatment recommended for score ≥9 and considered if =8

assess the risk of pathologic fracture. Table 8.4 illustrates the scoring system developed by Mirels to assign a score to a metastatic bone tumor to predict risk of fracture [8]. Not surprisingly, lesions that are larger, more painful, and associated with bony destruction have a higher risk of fracture and therefore warrant prophylactic treatment. Prophylactic treatment is preferred compared to treatment of a pathologic fracture because of decreased morbidity, decreased surgical time and blood loss, lower postoperative opioid requirements, improved rehab potential, and a higher rate of discharge to home versus a facility.

Mechanical load of the involved area must be considered when determining precautions. The proximal femur is the most common site of mechanical failure under continuous axial and torsional stresses. Sixty-five percent of all fractures that require surgery are in the femur. When the fracture involves the femoral head or neck, bone resection and prosthetic replacement is the preferred treatment. Although not a "weight bearing bone," the humerus is at high risk of fracture because of rotational forces from muscle. The decision to use an intramedullary nail is based on prognosis of the primary disease process, longer postoperative survival is the most important risk factor for eventual implant failure.

An ambulatory aid is recommended when there is activity-related pain and a radiographic lesion. A cane, crutches, or a walker can be prescribed depending on the functional status and comorbidities of the patient. Protected weight bearing should continue until fracture union.

Primary Bone and Soft Tissue Tumors

Primary malignant bone and soft tissue tumors are far less common than metastatic disease to bone. Table 8.5 characterizes common primary bone and soft tissue malignancies including characteristic location, age group, metastatic potential, survivorship, and treatment.

There are also benign bone tumors that may behave in a locally aggressive fashion and can even metastasize [16]. Giant cell tumor of the bone can form a locally destructive lytic lesion typically in the metaphyseal region of long bones, occurring commonly around the joint (particularly the knee) [17]. Giant cell tumors may also metastasize to lungs, so workup must include imaging of the lungs. Treatment usually involves intralesional curettage and removal of tumor tissue from the bone. Typically, adjuvant treatment within the void left after tumor resection in the form of liquid nitrogen, phenol, or argon beam can be used to fully eradicate tumor tissue and decrease risk of recurrence. Often the cavity that remains after curettage of giant cell tumor of bone must be replaced with allograft/autograft bone or cement augmentation with supplemental fixation. Therefore, rehabilitation after treatment of this tumor is similar to fracture care, as weight bearing is often restricted. Focus on maintaining joint range of motion (both actively and passively) is crucial postoperatively. Systemic treatment in the form of denosumab (monoclonal antibody against RANKL) can be used in disease where tumor is in a location that precludes adequate resection [18].

Posttreatment surveillance of orthopedic tumors is somewhat dependent on the histologic grade of the tumor. In

TABLE 8.5 Primary bone and soft tissue malignancies [9–15]

Tumor	Location	Age group	Metastatic potential	Survivorship	Treatment
Ewing's sarcoma	Diaphysis of long bones	Age 5–25	Lungs most common site	70% for localized disease 30% for metastatic at 5 years	Neoadjuvant chemo – surgical resection – adjuvant chemo ± radiation
Osteosarcoma	Metaphysis of long bones (most common distal femur)	Ages 10–14 Age > 60	Lungs most common site	60–78% for localized disease 20–30% for metastatic at 5 years	Neoadjuvant chemo – surgical resection – adjuvant chemo
Chondrosarcoma	Pelvis, proximal humerus, proximal/distal femur	Age > 40	Higher grade = greater metastatic potential	83% for Grade I conventional 28% for dedifferentiated at 10 years	Surgery only (does not respond to chemo/radiation)

(continued)

TABLE 8.5 (continued)

Tumor	Location	Age group	Metastatic potential	Survivorship	Treatment
Liposarcoma	Lower extremity	Age > 50	More commonly extrapulmonary	Dependent on subtype, 50% survival for high grade at 5 years	Surgery ± radiation
Rhabdomyosarcoma	Extremities, GU system, head/neck	Age < 20	Bone marrow and nodal mets most common	Age dependent, 27% in adults, 61% in children at 5 years	Surgery ± chemo and radiation
Synovial sarcoma	Near (not within) joints of shoulder, knee, elbow, foot	Age < 30	Lungs most common site	60% at 5 years	Surgery + radiation ± chemo

general, the American College of Radiology recommends follow-up imaging every 3–6 months for the first 5 years post resection and moving the interval to every 6–12 months after the first 5 years [19]. This may include MRI of the primary tumor site and CT of chest for lesions that metastasize to lungs.

Radiation

Metastatic disease to bone is often treated with radiation for palliation of bone pain regardless of cancer type. Radiation therapy can be used alone or in combination with surgery and/or chemotherapy. Types of radiation include external beam radiation therapy, stereotactic techniques, and brachytherapy. Adverse effects vary with the type of radiation and the tissue exposed. Early side effects may include soft tissue swelling, skin changes, nausea, fatigue, and low blood counts [20]. Diarrhea and infertility may occur (if pelvis or abdomen in field). Late side effects include radiation-induced cancer, fractures, and radiation fibrosis, which can affect nerves and/or muscles causing weakness and stiffness [21]. (See Radiation fibrosis chapter.)

Bisphosphonates and denosumab delay complications, relieve symptoms, and improve quality of life. Zoledronic acid (ZA) is the most effective bisphosphonate for the prevention of morbidity. Denosumab is more effective than ZA for the prevention of skeletal morbidity from solid tumors. The use of bisphosphonates in women depends on whether the patient is of childbearing age since these medications do cross the placenta. Treating the primary cancer is of utmost importance, and this will vary widely on the type and stage of disease.

Symptomatic multiple myeloma is treated by hematopoietic cell transplantation (HCT) and/or chemotherapy depending on eligibility and risk stratification [22]. Dexamethasone may be used as an adjunct treatment in myeloma patients ineligible for HCT or patients with metastatic disease getting radiation. This can also adversely affect bone health.

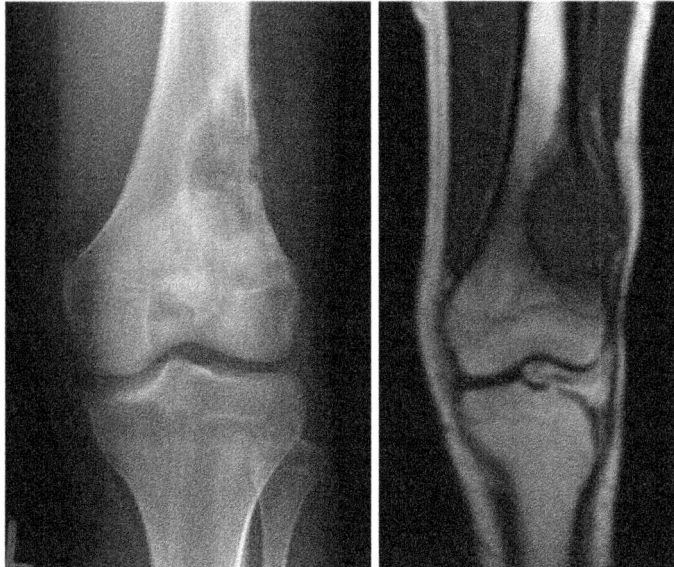

FIGURE 8.1   Radiographs and MRI of distal femoral lesion

Case Example

A 16-year-old male presented with 2 months of nonspecific left knee pain. Knee radiographs taken by his pediatrician showed a destructive lesion in the distal femoral metaphysis. MRI and oncologic workup was done, which confirmed localized disease (Fig. 8.1). Incisional biopsy was done, confirming diagnosis of osteosarcoma. Because of the extraarticular nature of the lesion, limb salvage surgery was indicated. After neoadjuvant chemotherapy, he underwent excision of the tumor and reconstruction with a distal femur replacement (Fig. 8.2). He remains disease free at 3 years postoperatively.

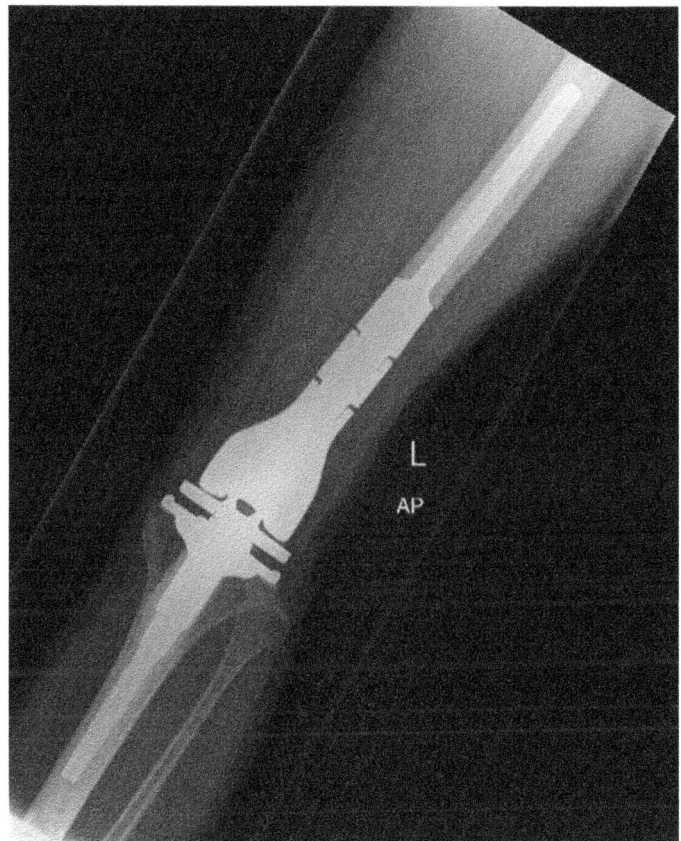

FIGURE 8.2 Appearance after surgical fixation

Conclusion

Musculoskeletal tumors comprise a heterogeneous mix of pathology affecting multiple age groups and anatomic locations. Understanding how these tumors are treated allows for a comprehensive rehabilitation plan. Fortunately, advances in technology have improved survival and function after treatment.

Multiple Choice Questions

1. A 40-year-old male is diagnosed with metastatic bone lesion from prostate cancer. What is the typical appearance?

    A. Blastic
    B. Lytic
    C. Mixed
    D. Both A and B

2. Which of the following amputation levels is associated with greatest increase in energy expenditure compared to baseline?

    A. Short BKA
    B. Syme
    C. AKA
    D. Bilateral BKA

3. All of the following tumors are radiation sensitive EXCEPT?

    A. Breast
    B. Chondrosarcoma
    C. Prostate
    D. Ewing's Sarcoma

4. A 74-year-old female with a history of lung cancer is seen in clinic. She complains of pain with ambulation and hip motion and has difficulty bearing weight on her right leg. She is found to have a lytic metastasis to the proximal femur involving 50% of the bone width. Based on the Mirels scoring system, what would be her score and recommended treatment?

    A. 6 – prophylactic surgery
    B. 6 – nonoperative treatment

C. 7 – nonoperative treatment
D. 10 – prophylactic surgery

5. An 80-year-old male is found to have a lytic lesion of the femur and undergoes a biopsy. He has no history of malignancy. Which tumor type is most likely to be seen on histology?

A. Chondrosarcoma
B. Osteosarcoma
C. Metastatic solid organ tumor
D. Giant cell tumor of bone

Answers

1. A
2. D
3. B
4. D lower ext (2) + lytic (3) + one half (2) + functional pain (3)
5. C

References

1. Enneking WF. Musculoskeletal tumor surgery. New York: Churchill Livingstone; 1983.
2. Katsanos K, Sabharwal T, Adam A. Percutaneous cementoplasty. Semin Intervent Radiol. 2010;27(2):137–47.
3. Waters RL, Perry J, Antonelli D, Hislop H. Energy cost of walking of amputees: the influence of level of amputation. J Bone Joint Surg Am. 1976;58(1):42–6.
4. Local Coverage Determination (LCD): Lower Limb Prostheses (L33787). Centers for Medicare and Medicaid Services.
5. Mundy GR. Metastasis to bone: causes, consequences and therapeutic opportunities. Nat Rev Cancer. 2002;2(8):584–93.
6. Quinn RH, Randall RL, Benevenia J, Berven SH, Raskin KA. Contemporary management of metastatic bone disease: tips and tools of the trade for general practitioners. J Bone Joint Surg Am. 2013;95(20):1887–95.

7. Greenspan A, Jundt G, Remagen W. Differential diagnosis in orthopaedic oncology. Philadelphia: Lippincott Williams & Wilkins; 2007.
8. Mirels H. Metastatic disease in long bones. A proposed scoring system for diagnosing impending pathologic fractures. Clin Orthop Relat Res. 1989;249:256–64.
9. Durfee RA, Mohammed M, Luu HH. Review of osteosarcoma and current management. Rheumatol Ther. 2016;3(2):221–43. Epub 2016 Oct 19.
10. Ozaki T. Diagnosis and treatment of Ewing sarcoma of the bone: a review article. J Orthop Sci. 2015;20(2):250–63.
11. Kridis WB, Toumi N, Chaari H, et al. A review of Ewing sarcoma treatment: is it still a subject of debate? Rev Recent Clin Trials. 2017;12(1):19–23.
12. Nassif NA, Tseng W, Borges C, Chen P, Eisenberg B. Recent advances in the management of liposarcoma. F1000Res. 2016;5:2907.
13. Gelderblom H, Hogendoorn PC, Dijkstra SD, et al. The clinical approach towards chondrosarcoma. Oncologist. 2008;13(3):320–9.
14. Egas-bejar D, Huh WW. Rhabdomyosarcoma in adolescent and young adult patients: current perspectives. Adolesc Health Med Ther. 2014;5:115–25.
15. Stacchiotti S, Van Tine BA. Synovial sarcoma: current concepts and future perspectives. J Clin Oncol. 2018;36(2):180–7.
16. Hakim DN, Pelly T, Kulendran M, Caris JA. Benign tumours of the bone: a review. J Bone Oncol. 2015;4(2):37–41.
17. Sobti A, Agrawal P, Agarwala S, Agarwal M. Giant cell tumor of bone – an overview. Arch Bone Joint Surg. 2016;4(1):2–9.
18. Xu SF, Adams B, Yu XC, Xu M. Denosumab and giant cell tumour of bone-a review and future management considerations. Curr Oncol. 2013;20(5):e442–7.
19. Roberts CC, et al. ACR appropriateness criteria on metastatic bone disease. J Am College Radiol. 2010;7(6):400–9.
20. Mitin T, Loeffler JS, Vora SR. Radiation therapy techniques in cancer treatment. Last updated 1 Aug 2017. https://www.uptodate.com/contents/radiation-therapy-techniques-in-cancer-treatment.
21. Rajkumar SV, Kyle RA, Connor RF. Overview of the management of multiple myeloma. Last updated 19 July 2018. https://www.uptodate.com/contents/multiple-myeloma-overview-of-management.
22. Stubblefield MD. Neuromuscular complications of radiation therapy. Muscle Nerve. 2017;56(6):1031–40.

Chapter 9
Cancer of the Respiratory and Intrathoracic Organs

Charles Mitchell, Vishwa Raj, and Terrence Pugh

Introduction

Lung cancer is one of the most common oncological diagnoses in the USA. Several different pathologies exist, but all are associated with significant medical comorbidities with functional implications. The purpose of this chapter is to review the most common diagnoses of lung cancer, treatment options, and opportunities for rehabilitative intervention.

C. Mitchell (✉) · V. Raj · T. Pugh
Oncology Rehabilitation at Carolinas Rehabilitation of Atrium Health, Charlotte, NC, USA

Cancer Rehabilitation Section of Rehabilitation Department of Supportive Care at Levine Cancer Institute, Charlotte, NC, USA
e-mail: Charles.Mitchell@atriumhealth.org;
Vishwa.Raj@atriumhealth.org; Terrence.Pugh@atriumhealth.org

© Springer Nature Switzerland AG 2020   127
J. Baima, A. Khanna (eds.), *Cancer Rehabilitation*,
https://doi.org/10.1007/978-3-030-44462-4_9

Pathology

The American Cancer Society's Surveillance Research esti-mates the number of new cases of lung and bronchus cancer in 2018 to be 234,030. The median age of lung cancer diagno-sis in the USA is 70 years [1]. Lung cancer is frequently diag-nosed in its later stages, possibly due to a delayed presentation with overlapping cardiopulmonary symptoms related to smoking, such as cough or dyspnea. Moreover, almost 40% of patients diagnosed with early-stage lung cancer are not surgi-cal candidates due to comorbidities related to smoking, such as FEV1 <40% [2]. People at high risk for lung cancer include those with a history of cigarette smoking and second-hand exposure, as well as occupational hazards including asbestos, beryllium, uranium, or radon. Screening high-risk individuals for lung cancer with a low-dose CT chest can reduce mortal-ity by 20% [3].

Small cell lung cancer (SCLC) represents nearly 13% of lung cancer cases in the USA and is strongly associated with smoking. Without mediastinal lymph nodal involvement, SCLC patients are rarely surgical candidates. Prophylactic cranial irradiation offers a modest improvement to the 5-year survival rate due to a high risk of brain metastasis [4]. For early-stage SCLC, thoracic radiotherapy given alongside che-motherapies can provide cure in about 30% of patients [5]. However, almost two-thirds of patients diagnosed with SCLC are already advance stage requiring palliative treatment goals. Platinum-based chemotherapy has an initial response rate of almost 70%, but disease recurrence is common and develops in a median time of 4–5 months. If relapse occurs after 3 months patients are considered "sensitive" and are offered salvage therapy to promote a period of progression-free survival. For example, administration of topotecan has a response rate of 20%. It is one of the few agents to demonstrate clinical benefit, but it does not improve overall survival [6]. The median survival rate for advanced-stage SCLC is less than a year with treatment and less than 2 months without treatment [7].

Non-small cell lung cancers (NSCLC) include adenocarcinoma, squamous cell carcinoma, and large cell carcinoma. Adenocarcinoma is the most common subtype of lung cancer, representing around 40% of all cases. Adenocarcinoma is typically located in the lung periphery and results in distal metastases to lymph and brain tissue. Never-smokers who develop lung cancer most frequently present with adenocarcinoma. Squamous cell carcinoma is centrally located and associated with hypercalcemia. Patients typically have a smoking history, but the incidence is decreasing within the USA because of tobacco cessation [8]. Large cell carcinoma represents <5% of NSCLC and is strongly associated with a smoking history [9]. It has an aggressive clinical course and poor survival rates even with early-stage disease.

NSCLC is treated according to stage. If diagnosed in the early-stages, surgical resection or occasionally stereotactic radiation are curative. Localized lung cancers can be resected with lobectomy, pneumonectomy, or sleeve resection removing tumor and bronchus [10]. The overall 5-year survival for all patients diagnosed with NSCLC is less than 20%. Adjuvant chemotherapies are used in stage II and III disease after surgical resection due to the high risk of metastasis [11, 12]. NSCLC diagnosed as stage IV are treated with palliative measures. Surgical resection of tumors beyond stage III is controversial, but radiotherapy can be considered curative for stage III and palliative for stage IV disease. In advanced-stage NSCLC, systemic chemotherapy can improve quality of life and modestly improve survival. Standard chemotherapy is typically platinum-based with a response rate of 20% and a median survival of about 9 months [13, 14]. Radiation therapy is reserved for palliation of symptoms from metastasis, such as painful bone lesions, neurological dysfunction from brain lesions, or obstructive lung disease because of lesions to the bronchus or superior vena cava.

Mesothelioma is uncommon with an incidence of less than 3000 cases annually in the USA [15]. Mesothelioma typically occurs in the pleura, but can also occur in the pericardium or peritoneum. The major risk factor for mesothelioma is exposure to asbestos with a latency period of 40 years before presentation of the cancer [16]. Median age at diagnosis is 63 years with median survival of stages I-IV ranging from 21 months to 12 months [17]. Clinical symptoms can include dyspnea from a pleural effusion or pain from tumor invasion of the pleura. Diagnosis of mesothelioma can be positive in pleural fluid, needle biopsy, and thoracoscopic biopsy up to 60%, 86%, and 98%, respectively [18]. Staging is performed with CT of the abdomen and pelvis with contrast, as well as a PET-CT. Although most patients present with advanced-stage disease, those diagnosed in early stages are amenable to multimodal treatment. Surgery alone can provide a median survival of 11 months. Median survival increases to 20 months with surgery and chemotherapy or radiation [17].

Common Impairments

- Pain
- Dyspnea
- Fatigue
- Cognition
- Sleep/wake cycle
- Quality of life
- Comorbid COPD
- Radiation fibrosis
- Chemotherapy-induced peripheral neuropathy

Patients who have been treated for lung cancer may present with a variety of impairments during evaluation by a physiatrist at the acute care consultation, inpatient rehabilitation admission, or outpatient clinic appointment. Common medical considerations associated this diagnosis include antibiotics for pneumonia, oxygen needs after treatment for a pleural effusion, palliative radiation for a painful bone metastasis, or a painful pleural injury after a tumor biopsy. Patients frequently have limited exercise tolerance from dyspnea and pain. A history of tobacco use may lead to comorbidities, such as COPD, cardiac dysfunction, and stroke.

Chronic smokers are more likely to develop postoperative pulmonary complications from impaired sputum clearance and inability to breathe deeply or cough due to pain associated with surgery. However, improvement of postoperative pain tolerance is possible if patients stop smoking at least 3 weeks before surgery [19].

Surgical procedures for diagnosis and treatment can result in significant impairment. Although respiratory muscle weakness is not as prominent in patients undergoing video-assisted thoracic surgical (VATS) procedures, it remains a significant source of postoperative pain [20]. For NSCLC, functional decline after lobectomy or pneumonectomy is manifested as increased dyspnea, worsening exercise capacity, diminished physical functioning, and pain [21]. Pain after surgery can be present in 90% of patients up to 6 years later [22].

Chest wall radiation therapy can cause fibrosis, pleural pain, pneumonitis, dermatitis, and esophagitis [23]. Radiation fibrosis can present immediately during the acute phase of therapy, within 3 months in the early-delayed phase of therapy, or after 3 months in the late-delayed phase of therapy [24]. The benefits of radiation therapy often outweigh the risks in patients with unresectable tumors when treating intrathoracic malignancies. It can also reduce pain and skeletal-related events in asymptomatic bone disease [25]. Rehabilitation interventions can aid in pain reduction to improve functional outcomes [21]. Active breathing coordination may help keep the tumor in the radiation treatment field and minimize the risk of damaging healthy tissue including the heart [26, 27].

Chemotherapy may be prescribed to patients concurrent with surgery or radiation therapy. Platinum-based chemotherapies, such as cisplatin [28] and oxaliplatin [29], may result in chemotherapy-induced peripheral neuropathy (CIPN) in up to 85–95% of patients [24]. Newer treatment regimens, such as nab-Paclitaxel plus carboplatin, have been shown to have better side effect profiles and reduced rates of CIPN [30]. CIPN may cause painful sensory changes in the hands and feet, which can impair sleep and participation with exercise. This can also result in proprioceptive changes, and motor weakness impacts functional independence.

Impaired feeding, eating, walking, breathing, and sleep can occur throughout the treatment spectrum [31]. In early-stage NSCLC, impaired quality of life (QOL) results from a decline in physical function, general health, vitality, sexual function, and mental health [32]. Lung cancer survivors additionally reported a decrease in health-related QOL. However, exercise therapies can improve physical function and overall well-being. The POSITIVE study demonstrated that patients with inoperable advanced-stage lung cancer improved their physical functioning, fatigue, muscle strength/endurance, immunity, and overall well-being with an exercise program and interval phone calls from a care manager [33].

Evidence for Exercise Throughout Spectrum of Care

Patients with lung cancer can use exercise and physical and occupational therapy throughout the course of their disease to help reduce morbidity and improve their quality of life. The American Cancer Society (ACS) advises patients to be physically active during their cancer treatments to prevent muscle wasting, reduce treatment side effects, and improve overall fitness [34]. Activities should be tailored to the individual based on the type and stage of cancer, timing with cancer treatment, and premorbid physical fitness level. Prior to starting any exercise program, patients should consult with their physicians. Uncontrolled pain, nausea, or vomiting as well as significant anemia, thrombocytopenia, leukopenia, or electrolyte abnormalities should be addressed to optimize safety with activities. To promote activity tolerance, physicians can additionally target specific components of physical disability via impairment-driven rehabilitation. Impairments that frequently limit activity tolerance include mobility, pain, dyspnea, and fatigue [35].

Presurgical physical therapy or unimodal prehabilitation has been demonstrated to reduce hospital stay and postoperative complication rates. Using a 4-week prehabilitation pulmonary program, individuals had shorter length of stay and shorter duration of chest tubes compared to the control group, who used breathing exercises only [36]. Because post-surgical patients demonstrate reduced exercise tolerance and reduced peak oxygen consumption [37], a structured physical therapy program could help improve their morbidity. Significant improvement on pulmonary function tests and peak oxygen consumption is also noted with exercise [38].

Patients with inoperable lung cancer who are receiving chemotherapies may also benefit from exercise therapies. Significant improvement to physiologic and emotional quality of life measures is noted for Stage III and IV lung cancer patients who completed aerobic exercise training during chemotherapy [39]. Tai Chi has been found to reduce fatigue as measured by reduction of the Multidimensional Fatigue Symptoms Inventory-Short Form score for individuals receiving chemotherapy [40].

Home-based exercise programs have also been shown to be effective for patients with stage IV lung cancer to improve mobility, fatigue, and sleep quality [41]. Exercise modalities, such as pulmonary rehabilitation, aerobic exercise, resistance training, exercise balance programs, and Qi Gong, result in reduction of fatigue, dyspnea, and depression [42].

When patients progress to survivorship, physical activity may help reduce the risk of a second cancer or other chronic disease. The ACS recommends that cancer survivors avoid being sedentary by returning to normal daily activities as soon as possible when cleared by a physician. They specifically recommend regular aerobic exercise for at least 150 minutes per week and include strength training exercises at least 2 days per week [34].

Conclusion

Lung cancer diagnoses are very common in the USA. Providers should anticipate functional impairments associated with the diagnoses, as well as treatment effects. With appropriate rehabilitation interventions, individuals can improve functionality and overall QOL.

Case Study

A 79-year-old female presented with bilateral lower extremity edema and 2 months of progressive dyspnea on exertion. She was hypoxic on room air, placed on supplemental oxygen, and transported to a nearby emergency room for further evaluation. She was experiencing a nonproductive cough, poor appetite, and mild weight loss. She had a 10 pack-year history of cigarette smoking.

CT of the chest revealed a large right-sided pleural effusion, several pulmonary nodules, mediastinal lymphadenopathy, and a pericardial effusion. She was admitted the same day to the cardiology step-down unit. Transthoracic surgery performed a pericardial window and a thoracotomy. Chest tube was placed and drained 450 mL of serosanguinous fluid. The cytology was inconclusive for malignancy. Bronchoscopy with lavage was positive for adenocarcinoma of the lung. After her bronchoscopy she developed acute respiratory distress and was anticoagulated for pulmonary embolism diagnosed by CT angiogram. Medical oncology ordered a PET-CT, revealing hypermetabolic lesions in the liver, bone, and mediastinal and hilar lymph nodes (Fig. 9.1), and diagnosed her with stage IV lung cancer. Radiation oncology recommended 10 fractions to her right hilum and mediastinum prior to initiation of chemotherapy.

Physiatry evaluated the patient for function, care coordination, and disposition planning. Medical complexity affecting functional status included acute pulmonary embolism, cancer burden of the lungs and lymphatic system, pleural effusion, new oxygen requirement, and generalized deconditioning. Prior to inpatient rehabilitation admission, physical therapy documented gait status at minimum-assist with a rolling walker for 100 feet with several rest breaks due to decreased endurance and shortness of breath.

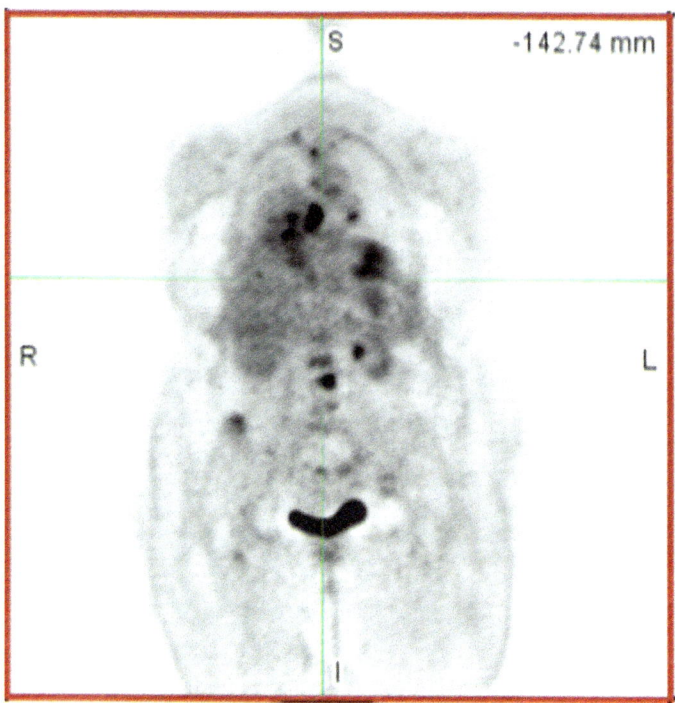

FIGURE 9.1 PET-CT revealing hypermetabolic lesions to the right lung, liver, L4 vertebral body, right iliac bone, and mediastinal and hilar lymph nodes, as well as innumerable subcentimeter pulmonary nodules consistent with lymphangitic spread of tumor

The patient made gradual functional improvements at rehabilitation. Her sleep was impaired due to orthopnea and she was unable to wean off oxygen. A repeat chest X-ray revealed reaccumulation of her right-sided pleural effusion (Fig. 9.2) and she had a PleurX catheter placed for expected reaccumulation and daily drainage of recurrent malignant effusion. Improvement was noted after repeat chest X-ray (Fig. 9.3). Her catheter volumes stabilized at 200 mL daily. The daughter completed family education for assistance with

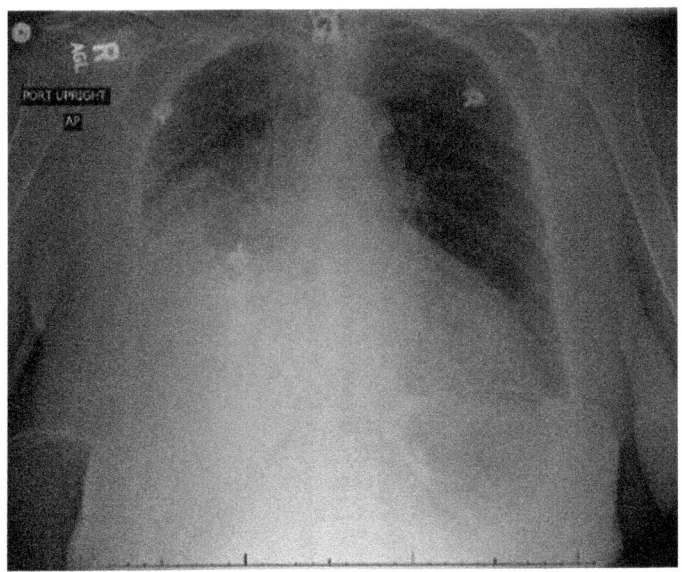

FIGURE 9.2 Chest X-ray revealing a recurrent right-sided pleural effusion

PleurX drainage, as well as safety with ambulation and trans-fers. She continued to require supplemental oxygen 2 L per nasal cannula to maintain oxygen saturations above 88% during physical exertion. Her rehab discharge therapy evalu-ations improved to modified independent for all ADLs, including completing a 6-minute walk test with over 400 feet using a rolling walker. The patient was safely discharged to home in good functional condition with intermittent supervi-sion from family available. She had close follow-up planned with medical oncology to repeat CT imaging after comple-tion of radiation therapy, and to consider palliative chemo-therapy given her improvement in functional status. When followed by physiatry 6 weeks later, she continued 2 L sup-plemental oxygen per nasal cannula and daily drainage of her PleurX catheter. The patient denied any recent falls,

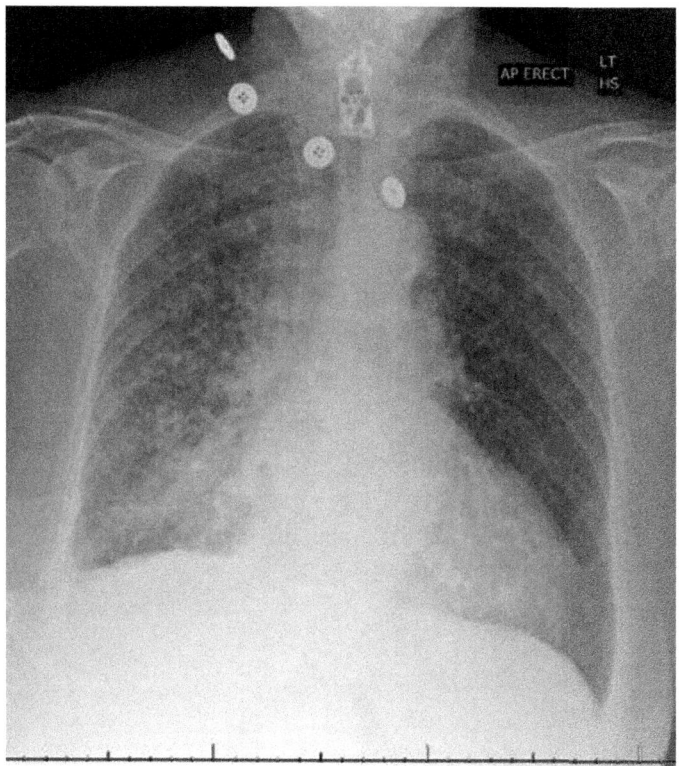

FIGURE 9.3 Chest X-ray revealing a significant decrease in right-sided pleural effusion s/p placement of a PleurX catheter. Additionally, there is diffuse interstitial nodular pattern within the lungs which is suspicious for lymphangitic spread of malignancy

reported confidence with car transfers, and continued to perform all ADLs modified independent, including ambulation with a rolling walker. She was deemed appropriate for transition to outpatient therapies for higher-level balance and further energy conservation strategies given her upcoming palliative chemotherapy plan.

Multiple Choice Questions

1. The American Cancer Society's Surveillance Research estimates the number of new cases of lung and bronchus cancer in 2018 to be:

   A. 2030
   B. 23,030
   C. 234,030
   D. 2,340,030

2. The most common subtype of lung cancer is:

   A. Mesothelioma
   B. Adenocarcinoma
   C. Squamous cell carcinoma
   D. Large cell carcinoma

3. The latency period from exposure to development of mesothelioma is estimated to be:

   A. 4 months
   B. 4 years
   C. 40 months
   D. 40 years

4. Nonsmokers who develop lung cancer most frequently develop:

   A. Mesothelioma
   B. Adenocarcinoma
   C. Squamous cell carcinoma
   D. Large cell carcinoma

5. The American Cancer Society advises patients to be physically active during their cancer treatments to:

   A. Prevent muscle wasting
   B. Reduce treatment side effects
   C. Improve overall fitness
   D. All the above

Answers

1. C
2. B
3. D
4. B
5. D

References

1. Owonikoko TK, Ragin CC, Belani CP, et al. Lung cancer in elderly patients: an analysis of the surveillance, epidemiology, and end results database. J Clin Oncol. 2007;25:5570–7.
2. Brunelli A, Kim AW, Berger KI, Adrizzo-Harris DJ. Physiologic evaluation of the patient with lung cancer being considered for resectional surgery: diagnosis and management of lung cancer, 3rd ed. American College of Chest Physicians evidence-based clinical practice guidelines. Chest. 2013;143:e166S–90S.
3. National Lung Screening Trial Research Team, Aberle DR, Adams AM, et al. Reduced lung-cancer mortality with low-dose computed tomographic screening. N Engl J Med. 2011;365:395–409.
4. Le Pechoux C, Dunant A, Senan S, et al. Standard-dose versus higher-dose prophylactic cranial irradiation in patients with limited-stage small-cell lung cancer in complete remission after chemotherapy and thoracic radiotherapy: a randomised clinical trial. Lancet Oncol. 2009;10:467–74.
5. Turrisi AT, Kim K, Blum R, et al. Twice-daily compared with once-daily thoracic radiotherapy in limited small-cell lung cancer treated concurrently with cisplatin and etoposide. N Engl J Med. 1999;340:265–71.
6. O'Brien ME, Ciuleanu TE, Tsekov H, et al. Phase III trial comparing supportive care alone with supportive care with oral topotecan in patients with relapsed small-cell lung cancer. J Clin Oncol. 2006;24:5441–7.
7. Kalemkerian GP, Akerley W, Bogner P, et al. Small cell lung cancer. J Natl Compr Cancer Netw. 2013;11:78–98.
8. Sterlacci W, Savic S, Schmid T, et al. Tissue-sparing application of the newly proposed IASLC/ATS/ERS classification of

adenocarcinoma of the lung shows practical diagnostic and prognostic impact. Am J Clin Pathol. 2012;137:946–56.

9. Paci M, Cavazza A, Annessi V, et al. Large cell neuroendocrine carcinoma of the lung: a 10-year clinicopathologic retrospective study. Ann Thorac Surg. 2004;77:1163.

10. Predina JD, Kunkala M, Aliperti LA, Singhal AK, Singhal S. Sleeve lobectomy: current indications and future directions. Ann Thorac Cardiovasc Surg. 2010;16:310–8.

11. Pignon JP, Tribodet H, Scagliotti GV, et al. Lung adjuvant cisplatin evaluation: a pooled analysis by LACE Collaborative Group. J Clin Oncol. 2008;26:3552–9.

12. Strauss GM, Wang XF, Maddaus M, et al. Adjuvant chemotherapy in stage IB non-small cell lung cancer (NSCLC): long-term follow-up of Cancer and Leukemia Group B (CALGB) 9633. J Clin Oncol. 2011;29:7015.

13. Spiro SG, Rudd RM, Souhami RL, et al. Chemotherapy versus supportive care in advanced non-small cell lung cancer: improved survival without detriment to quality of life. Thorax. 2004;59:828–36.

14. Sandler A, Gray R, Perry MC, et al. Paclitaxel-carboplatin alone or with bevacizumab for non-small-cell lung cancer. N Engl J Med. 2006;355(24):2542–50.

15. Price B, Ware A. Time trend of mesothelioma incidence in the United States and projection of future cases: an update based on SEER data for 1973-2005. Crit Rev Toxicol. 2009;39(7):576–88.

16. Robinson B. Malignant pleural mesothelioma: an epidemiological perspective. Ann Cardiothorac Surg. 2012;1(4):491–6.

17. Rusch VW, Giroux D, Kennedy C, et al. Initial analysis of the international association for the study of lung cancer mesothelioma database. J Thorac Oncol. 2012;7(11):1631–9.

18. Adams RF, Gleeson FV. Percutaneous image-guided cutting-needle biopsy of the pleura in the presence of a suspected malignant effusion. Radiology. 2001;219(2):510–4.

19. Zhao S, Chen F, Wang D, et al. Effect of preoperative smoking cessation on postoperative pain outcomes in elderly patients with high nicotine dependence. Medicine (Baltimore). 2019;98(3):e14209. https://doi.org/10.1097/MD.0000000000014209.

20. Kendall F, Abreu P, Pinho J, et al. The role of physiotherapy in patients undergoing pulmonary surgery for lung cancer: a literature review. Rev Port Pneumol. 2017;23(6):343–51. https://doi.org/10.1016/j.rppnen/2017.05.003. Accessed 1/14/19.

21. Smith SR, Khanna A, Wisotzky EM. An evolving role for cancer rehabilitation in the era of low-dose lung computed tomography screening. PMR. 2017;9:S407–14.
22. Iyer S, Roughley A, Rider A, et al. The symptom burden of non-small cell lung cancer in the USA: a real-world cross-sectional study. Support Care Cancer. 2014;22:181–7.
23. Chen J, Lu JJ, Ma N, et al. Early stage non-small cell lung cancer treated with pencil beam scanning particle therapy: retrospective analysis of early results on safety and efficacy. Radiat Oncol. 2019;14(1):16. https://doi.org/10.1186/s13014-019-1216-1.
24. New P. Radiation injury to the nervous system. Curr Opin Neurol. 2001;14:725–34.
25. Shulman RM, Meyer JE, Li T, Howell KJ. External beam radiation therapy (EBRT) for asymptomatic bone metastases in patients with solid tumors reduces the risk of skeletal-related events (SREs). Ann Palliat Med. 2018. pii: apm.2018.10.04; https://doi.org/10.21037/apm.2018.10.04.
26. den Otter LA, Kaza E, Kierkels RGJ, et al. Reproducibility of the lung anatomy under active breathing coordinator control: dosimetric consequences for scanned proton treatment. Med Phys. 2018;45(12):5525–34.
27. Kaza E, Dunlop A, Panek R, et al. Lung volume reproducibility under ABC control and self-sustained breath holding. J Appl Clin Med Phys. 2017;18(2):154–62. https://doi.org/10.1002/acm2.12034.
28. Butts CA, Ding K, Seymour L, et al. Randomized phase III trial of vinorelbine plus cisplatin compared with observation in completely resected stage IB and II non-small-cell lung cancer: updated survival analysis of JBR-10. J Clin Oncol. 2010;28(1):29–34.
29. Cheng X, Huo J, Wang D, et al. Herbal medicine AC591 prevents oxaliplatin-induced peripheral neuropathy in animal model and cancer patients. Front Pharmacol. 2017;8:344.
30. Garja A, Karim NA, Mulford D, et al. nab-Paclitaxel–based therapy in underserved patient populations: the ABOUND.PS2 study in patients with NSCLC and a performance status of 2. Front Oncol. 2018;8(253) https://doi.org/10.3389/fonc.2018.00253.
31. Fodeh SJ, Lazenby M, Bai M, et al. Functional impairments as symptoms in the symptom cluster analysis of patients newly diagnosed with advanced cancer. J Pain Symptom Manag. 2013;46(4):500–10. https://doi.org/10.1016/j.jpainsymman.2012.09.011.

32. Ostroff JS, Krebs P, Coups EJ, et al. Health-related quality of life among early-stage, non-small cell, lung cancer survivors. Lung Cancer. 2011;71(1):103–8. https://doi.org/10.1016/j.lungcan.2010.04.011.
33. Wiskermann J, Hummler S, Diepold C, et al. POSITIVE study: physical exercise program in non-operable lung cancer patients undergoing palliative treatment. BMC Cancer. 2016;16:499.
34. American Cancer Society ACS Guidelines for Physical Activity and the Cancer Patient. [Accessed January 31, 2019]. Available from: https://www.cancer.org/treatment/survivorship-during-and-after-treatment/staying-active/physical-activity-and-the-cancer-patient.html.
35. Silver JK, Baima J, Mayer RS. Impairment-driven cancer rehabilitation: an essential component of quality care and survivorship. CA Cancer J Clin. 2013;63(5):295–317.
36. Morano MT, Araujo AS, Nascimento FB, et al. Preoperative pulmonary rehabilitation versus chest physical therapy in patients undergoing lung cancer resection: a pilot randomized controlled trial. Arch Phys Med Rehabil. 2013;94:53–8.
37. Jones LW, Peddle CJ, Eves ND, Haykowsky MJ, Courneya KS, Mackey JR, Joy AA, Kumar V, Winton TW, Reiman T. Cancer. 2007;110(3):590–8.
38. Divisi D, Di Francesco C, Di Leonardo G, Crisci R. Preoperative pulmonary rehabilitation in patients with lung cancer and chronic obstructive pulmonary disease. Eur J Cardiothorac Surg. 2013;43:293–6.
39. Quist M, Rorth M, Langer S, et al. Safety and feasibility of a combined exercise intervention for inoperable lung cancer patients undergoing chemotherapy: a pilot study. Lung Cancer. 2012;75:203–8.
40. Zhang LL, Wang SZ, Chen HL, Yuan AZ. Tai Chi exercise for cancer-related fatigue in patients with lung cancer undergoing chemotherapy: a randomized controlled trial. J Pain Symptom Manag. 2016;51(3):504–11.
41. Cheville AL, Kollasch J, Vandenberg J, et al. A home-based exercise program to improve function, fatigue, and sleep quality in patients with stage IV lung and colorectal cancer: a randomized controlled trial. J Pain Symptom Manag. 2013;45(5):811–21.
42. Henshall CL, Allin L, Aveyard H. A systematic review and narrative synthesis to explore the effectiveness of exercise-based interventions in improving fatigue, dyspnea, and depression in lung cancer survivors. Cancer Nurs. 2018;42(4):295–306. https://doi.org/10.1097/NCC.0000000000000605.

Chapter 10
Cancer of the Skin

Grigory Syrkin

Introduction

Skin cancer is the most common malignancy worldwide. In the United States, among the ten most common cancer diagnoses, malignant melanoma is the one most rapidly increasing in incidence. A cancer rehabilitation physiatrist is more likely to work with populations that are prone to rare skin cancers, such as Kaposi's sarcoma, angiosarcoma, and Merkel cell carcinoma. Beyond managing impairments from local and systemic skin cancer treatment, a cancer rehabilitation physiatrist can provide lasting impact by mitigating risk factors implicated in the development of skin cancer.

Epidemiology

The two broadest categories of skin neoplasms are (1) malignant melanoma (MM) and (2) keratinocyte carcinomas (KC), of which there are two subtypes – basal cell carcinoma (BCC) and squamous cell carcinoma (SqCC). In the United States, MM comprises 7% of all new cancer diagno-

G. Syrkin (✉)
Department of Neurology, Rehabilitation Medicine Service, Memorial Sloan Kettering Cancer Center, New York, NY, USA
e-mail: syrking@mskcc.org

© Springer Nature Switzerland AG 2020   143
J. Baima, A. Khanna (eds.), *Cancer Rehabilitation*,
https://doi.org/10.1007/978-3-030-44462-4_10

ses in men and 4% in women and represents the most rapidly increasing cancer diagnosis among the ten most common neoplasms [1, 2]. Despite its slow-growing nature, KC is estimated to consume about 4% of all cancer-related care costs in the United States, a number that is likely to grow, since its incidence is expected to rise. Furthermore, even in industrialized countries with near-universal access to healthcare, such as Germany and the UK, the incidence of KC is estimated to have risen 30% and is expected to double by 2030 [3, 4].

BCC is the single most prevalent skin neoplasm, comprising about 80% of KC, with a lifetime risk of 33-39% and 23-28% for Caucasian men and women in the USA, respectively [5]. SqCC makes up about 20% of KC cases, or about 1,000,000 new cases in the USA, with about 9000 deaths per year, a rate that almost quadrupled in the last 25 years [6]. MM is expected to affect about 96,500 Americans, causing approximately 7000 deaths. Merkel Cell Carcinoma (MCC) is a very rare skin neoplasm in the general population (estimated at about 1600 per year in the USA), but is much more common among immunosuppressed patients, such as those with lymphoproliferative malignancies, and is the second most common cause of death due to skin cancer [7]. Other rare skin neoplasms that may be more frequently encountered in cancer patients include Kaposi's sarcoma and angiosarcoma (particularly associated with chronic lymphedema).

Risk Factors

Ultraviolet (UV) radiation, both naturally occurring and associated with indoor tanning (IT), older age, fair skin, and immunosuppression have been implicated in the development of all skin neoplasms [2, 5, 6, 8, 9]. Several types of skin cancer have been linked to viral infections, such as human papilloma virus for SqCC, Merkel cell polyoma virus for MCC, and Herpes simplex virus-8 for Kaposi's sarcoma.

Smoking has been shown to double the risk of SqCC, worsen the prognosis of angiosarcomas, but produce no effect on the incidence of MM or BCC [10–12]. Metastatic potential of SqCC varies by site, with tumors that arise from nonhealing wounds or other areas of chronic inflammation having 26% incidence of metastases [6]. Unlike other major malignancies, leisure time physical activity does not appear to protect against skin cancer, most likely due to its relationship with UV [13].

The importance of photoprotection for the vulnerable population cannot be overstated – up to 40% of new SqCC could be prevented through appropriate use of sunscreen [6] and up to 7% of new MM, 5.2% of BCC, and 7.5% SqCC cases could be avoided by eliminating use of indoor tanning (IT) [8]. Furthermore, radiation recall phenomenon (painful erythema and/or eruption in the previously irradiated areas) following UV exposure is a well-recognized problem in the oncologic population, particularly among patients exposed to methotrexate, gemcitabine, etoposide, and taxanes. This warrants counseling regarding photoprotection [14, 15]. Educating patients at risk, such as those engaged in outdoor work, is especially important, as those groups are known to use appropriate photoprotection measures at lower rates [3].

Treatment and Related Impairments: Early Stages

Local excision with or without micrography (Mohs' surgery) is the primary treatment modality for most types of resectable skin cancer. Detailed discussion of all possible impairment scenarios is beyond the scope of this text. When evaluating a patient for problems potentially related to excision of a skin neoplasm, the treating cancer rehabilitation physiatrist should review the operative report (if available) with awareness of the local anatomy. The margins may range from 4–6 mm for early BCC and SqCC to 3 cm for MCC with surgical bed reaching underlying fascia or periosteum [5, 6, 9]. Additional donor site morbidity should be considered, if the skin defect requires grafting. In general, impairments can be related to impaired venous or lymphatic drainage, transection of cutaneous nerve trunks, or myofascial and tendinous adhesions due to local scarring.

Photodynamic therapy (PDT) for early (in situ) SqCC and BCC involves topical application of photosensitive agents, such as 5-aminolevulinic acid or methyl aminolevulinate (MAL), followed by exposure to specific UV wavelengths [6, 16]. Common impairments from PDT include local pain, photosensitivity, and dermatitis.

Treatment and Related Impairments: Advanced and Metastatic Disease

Metastatic and locally advanced skin cancers carried a very poor prognosis prior to the recent advances in immunotherapy [17]. Treatment of advanced and metastatic skin neoplasms typically included cytotoxic chemotherapy drugs (platinols, taxanes, alkylating agents, anthracyclines, and anti-metabolites), lymphadenectomy, and localized radiotherapy, producing significant systemic side effects and regional morbidity. Some of the commonly encountered local adverse effects include fibrosis, lymphedema, and nerve palsies with associated musculoskeletal problems. One example of this is winged scapula due to spinal accessory neuropathy following neck dissection. Careful review of operative and radiotherapy records must be undertaken to gain insight into potential treatment morbidity, as radiation doses can be high (66-70Gy) and extend up to 5 cm beyond the involved area [9]. Recent advances in immunotherapy, starting with approval of ipilimumab for MM in 2011 dramatically changed the prognosis for patients with advanced skin neoplasms.

Table 10.1 summarizes commonly used treatment modalities and related side effects.

TABLE 10.1 Skin cancer treatment modalities and adverse effects

Modality	Malignancy	Possible adverse effects
Photodynamic therapy	Actinic keratosis (precursor), in situ SqCC, thin BCC	Local photosensitivity reaction, incomplete diagnostic information
Mohs' micrographic surgery Standard surgical excision	All operable skin cancers	Surgical site morbidity, impaired distal venous or lymphatic drainage
Cryotherapy, electrodesiccation, and curettage	Low-risk BCC and SqCC	Incomplete diagnostic information, cannot be used with hair-bearing areas
Topical agents: imiquimod, 5-fluorouracil, ingenol mebutate, diclofenac, retinoids	Low-risk BCC and SqCC	Dermatitis, pruritus, rash, flu-like symptoms (diclofenac, imiquimod and ingenol mebutate), photosensitivity
5-Fluorouracil(5-FU)/ Cisplatin, 5-FU/ Carboplatin, Paclitaxel/ Carboplatin	Locally advanced or metastatic SqCC	Neutropenia, peripheral neuropathy (ganglionopathy), cardiac arrhythmias
Vismodegib, sonidegib	Locally advanced or metastatic BCC	Myalgia, dysgeusia, anorexia, fatigue (25% rate of serious adverse events) [18–20]
Cetuximab	Locally advanced or metastatic SqCC	Acneiform rash, fatigue, malaise, sensory neuropathy, xeroderma, diarrhea, hepatitis, neutropenia, infection [21, 22]
Cemiplimab (Approved 9/2018)		Diarrhea, fatigue, nausea, constipation and rash (29% rate of serious adverse events) [23]

(continued)

TABLE 10.1 (continued)

Modality	Malignancy	Possible adverse effects
Ipilimumab Pembrolizumab Nivolumab	Advance or metastatic MM, SqCC	Fatigue, musculoskeletal pain, colitis (diarrhea, perforation), hepatitis, pneumonitis (3-4%), endocrinopathies (15% rate of serious adverse events – more likely with combination therapy) [24]
Avelumab	MCC	
Vemurafenib Dabrafenib Encorafenib	BRAF-mutated MM	Arthralgia, fatigue, photosensitivity, rash, secondary SqCC [25]
Trametinib	MM	Fatigue, hypertension, vomiting, diarrhea [25]
Radiation therapy	Adjuvant or palliative treatment	Radiation fibrosis syndrome, lymphedema, nerve palsies

Case Presentation

The patient is a 76-year-old right-hand-dominant man with past medical history of hypertension, hypercholesterolemia, and mild to moderate spinal spondylosis. He has never smoked and is a retired pastor who resides in an assisted living facility. He was diagnosed with a malignant melanoma of the left dorsal forearm, initially resected in 2011. Four years later he was found to have local recurrence of the disease and ipsilateral arm swelling, prompting staging workup that revealed axillary, mediastinal, and paraaortic lymphadenopathy. He underwent repeat wide local excision, requiring skin graft coverage and was started on ipilimumab monotherapy with good initial response. Lymphedema of the affected extremity (Fig. 10.1) was managed with an off-the-shelf compression glove and a sleeve, prescribed by his primary care physician (PCP).

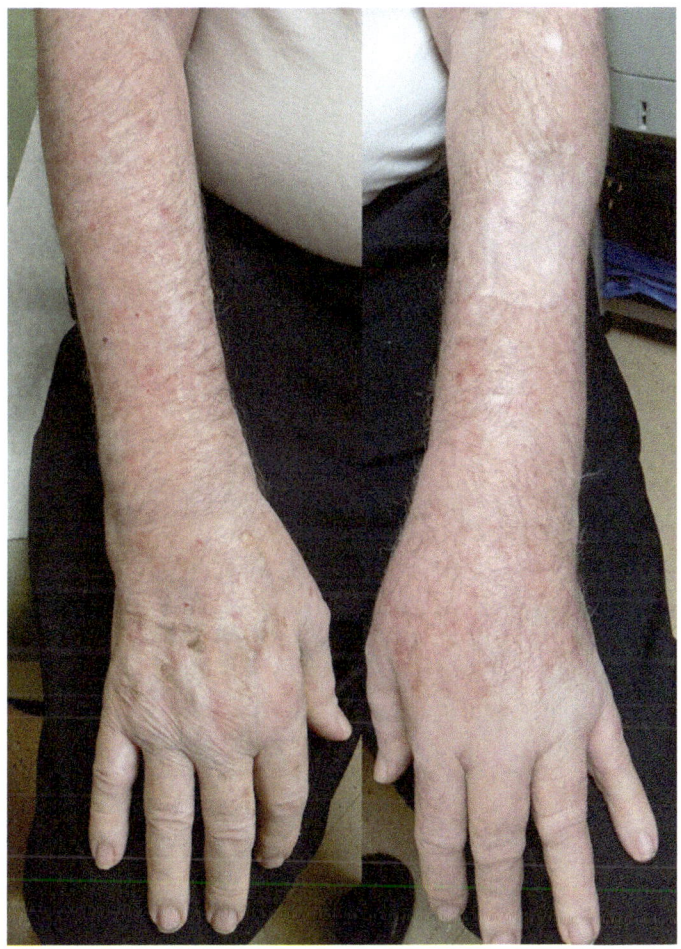

FIGURE 10.1 Gross appearance of the upper limbs, demonstrating good control of lymphedema in the affected (left) arm. Note well-healed surgical site with evidence of skin grafting

In late 2017 routine follow-up revealed progression of disease with involvement of right inguinal nodes, causing ipsilateral leg lymphedema (Fig. 10.2). He was started on nivolumab and after two treatments, was referred to physiatry for evaluation of right distal leg pain that precluded the patient

FIGURE 10.2 Gross appearance of the right lower leg, demonstrating adequate control of lymphedema and characteristic pes planus appearance

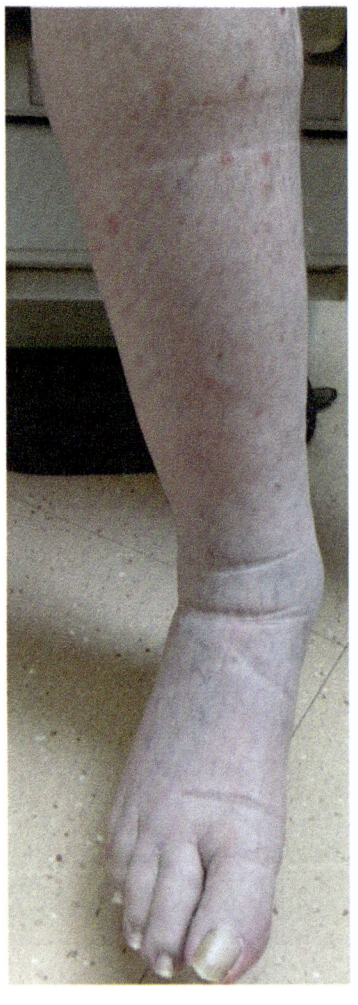

from taking his customary 2–3 hours walks. Physiatric evaluation revealed mildly symptomatic T6 compression fracture, mild proximal weakness, mild distal sensory loss to ankles, hip flexor and ankle plantarflexor contractures, pes planus, and significant tenderness along right tibialis posterior tendon, reproduced with both direct palpation and resisted foot inversion. Clinical diagnosis was tibialis posterior tendinopathy.

He was provided with footwear recommendations, home exercise program, an ankle foot orthotic prescription, and referred to physical therapy for lower limb stretching and ankle strengthening. Given the recent progression of disease, bony metastasis to right distal tibia was considered, but subsequently ruled out by the PET/CT. Initially, he responded well to the recommended care, but after two more cycles of nivolumab developed worsening right distal leg pain and more diffuse joint pains. He was lost to physiatric follow-up and transitioned to a manual wheelchair per his PCP. He was started on oral prednisone for presumed immune-mediated arthralgia due to nivolumab, which was subsequently held.

After notable improvement in joint pains, sustained by prednisone 5 mg PO daily, he resumed physiatric follow-up. He was found to have worsening of proximal weakness and progression of lower limb contractures. Interval imaging studies showed no bony metastatic lesions, stable T6 compression fracture, and progression of nodal disease, prompting his oncology team to resume nivolumab. He was advised to resume physical therapy and transition out of wheelchair as soon as possible to prevent further deconditioning, as neither his joint nor right ankle pain worsened during assisted ambulation during the office visit. His limb edema remained well controlled with compression garments and 4 weeks later he was navigating the community with a rolling walker. At 12-week follow-up, he demonstrated the ability to safely walk with close supervision and reported that his ambulation tolerance was approaching 20–30 minutes. He was advised to continue home exercise program, as well as supervised gait training at his assisted living facility.

Multiple Choice Questions

1. Which of the following skin neoplasms have been associated with indoor tanning bed use?

   A. Basal cell carcinoma
   B. Squamous cell carcinoma

    C. Malignant melanoma
    D. All of the above

2. Smoking is a modifiable risk factor for which of the following skin neoplasms?

    A. Basal cell carcinoma
    B. Squamous cell carcinoma
    C. Malignant melanoma
    D. All of the above

3. How much can appropriate sun protection reduce the risk
   of cutaneous squamous cell carcinoma?

    A. 10%
    B. 20%
    C. 30%
    D. 40%

4. Which of the following describes radiation recall phenomenon?

    A. Patients previously treated with methotrexate, gem-
       citabine, etoposide, and taxanes, experiencing painful
       erythema and/or eruption in the radiation treatment
       areas following UV or sunlight exposure
    B. Patients experiencing anxiety when describing their
       radiotherapy course
    C. Both a and b
    D. None of the above

5. Which of the following immune-mediated adverse events
   are most likely to be experienced by a patient receiving targeted immunotherapy for advanced malignant
   melanoma?

    A. Fatigue
    B. Musculoskeletal pain
    C. Pneumonitis
    D. Both a and b

Answers

1. D
   All of the above. Reference: O'Sullivan et al. [8].
2. B
   Squamous cell carcinoma. Reference: Dusingize et al [10].
3. D
   40%. Reference: Waldman and Schmults [6].
4. A
   Reference: Cohen [14], Sibaud et al. [15].
5. D
   Reference: Brahmer et al. [24], Luther et al. [25].

References

1. Siegel RL, Miller KD, Jemal A. Cancer statistics, 2019. CA Cancer J Clin. 2019;69(1):7–34.
2. Lazovich D, Vogel RI, Berwick M, Weinstock MA, Anderson KE, Warshaw EM. Indoor tanning and risk of melanoma: a case-control study in a highly exposed population. Cancer Epidemiol Biomark Prev. 2010;19(6):1557–68.
3. Zink A. Trends in the treatment and prevention of keratinocyte carcinoma (non-melanoma skin cancer). Curr Opin Pharmacol. 2019;46:19–23.
4. Nelson TG, Ashton RE. Low incidence of metastasis and recurrence from cutaneous squamous cell carcinoma found in a UK population: do we need to adjust our thinking on this rare but potentially fatal event? J Surg Oncol. 2017;116(6): 783–8.
5. Gandhi SA, Kampp J. Skin cancer epidemiology, detection, and management. Med Clin North Am. 2015;99(6): 1323–35.
6. Waldman A, Schmults C. Cutaneous squamous cell carcinoma. Hematol Oncol Clin North Am. 2019;33(1):1–12.
7. Ma JE, Brewer JD. Merkel cell carcinoma in immunosuppressed patients. Cancers (Basel). 2014;6(3):1328–50.

8. O'Sullivan DE, Brenner DR, Demers PA, et al. Indoor tanning and skin cancer in Canada: a meta-analysis and attributable burden estimation. Cancer Epidemiol. 2019;59:1–7.

9. Tello TL, Coggshall K, Yom SS, Yu SS. Merkel cell carcinoma: an update and review: current and future therapy. J Am Acad Dermatol. 2018;78(3):445–54.

10. Dusingize JC, Olsen CM, Pandeya NP, et al. Cigarette smoking and the risks of basal cell carcinoma and squamous cell carcinoma. J Invest Dermatol. 2017;137(8):1700–8.

11. Lee BL, Chen CF, Chen PC, et al. Investigation of prognostic features in primary cutaneous and soft tissue angiosarcoma after surgical resection: a retrospective study. Ann Plast Surg. 2017;78(3 Suppl 2):S41–6.

12. Dusingize JC, Olsen CM, Pandeya N, et al. Smoking and cutaneous melanoma: findings from the QSkin Sun and Health Cohort Study. Cancer Epidemiol Biomark Prev. 2018;27(8):874–81.

13. Moore SC, Lee IM, Weiderpass E, et al. Association of leisure-time physical activity with risk of 26 types of cancer in 1.44 million adults. JAMA Intern Med. 2016;176(6):816–25.

14. Cohen PR. Photodistributed erythema multiforme: paclitaxel-related, photosensitive conditions in patients with cancer. J Drugs Dermatol. 2009;8(1):61–4.

15. Sibaud V, Lebœuf NR, Roche H, et al. Dermatological adverse events with taxane chemotherapy. Eur J Dermatol. 2016;26(5):427–43.

16. Keyal U, Bhatta AK, Zhang G, Wang XL. Present and future perspectives of photodynamic therapy for cutaneous squamous cell carcinoma. J Am Acad Dermatol. 2019; 80(3):765–73. https://doi.org/10.1016/j.jaad.2018.10.042. Epub 2018 Oct 28.

17. Bridge JA, Lee JC, Daud A, Wells JW, Bluestone JA. Cytokines, chemokines, and other biomarkers of response for checkpoint inhibitor therapy in skin cancer. Front Med (Lausanne). 2018;5:351.

18. Lear JT, Migden MR, Lewis KD, et al. Long-term efficacy and safety of sonidegib in patients with locally advanced and metastatic basal cell carcinoma: 30-month analysis of the randomized phase 2 BOLT study. J Eur Acad Dermatol Venereol. 2018;32(3):372–81.

19. Ly P, Wolf K, Wilson J. A case of hepatotoxicity associated with vismodegib. JAAD Case Rep. 2019;5(1):57–9.

20. Sekulic A, Migden MR, Oro AE, et al. Efficacy and safety of vismodegib in advanced basal-cell carcinoma. N Engl J Med. 2012;366(23):2171–9.
21. Lu SM, Lien WW. Concurrent radiotherapy with cetuximab or platinum-based chemotherapy for locally advanced cutaneous squamous cell carcinoma of the head and neck. Am J Clin Oncol. 2018;41(1):95–9.
22. Que SKT, Zwald FO, Schmults CD. Cutaneous squamous cell carcinoma: management of advanced and high-stage tumors. J Am Acad Dermatol. 2018;78(2):249–61.
23. Migden MR, Rischin D, Schmults CD, et al. PD-1 blockade with cemiplimab in advanced cutaneous squamous-cell carcinoma. N Engl J Med. 2018;379(4):341–51.
24. Brahmer JR, Lacchetti C, Schneider BJ, et al. Management of immune-related adverse events in patients treated with immune checkpoint inhibitor therapy: American Society of Clinical Oncology clinical practice guideline. J Clin Oncol. 2018;36(17):1714.
25. Luther C, Swami U, Zhang J, Milhem M, Zakharia Y. Advanced stage melanoma therapies: detailing the present and exploring the future. Crit Rev Oncol/Hematol. 2019;133:99–111.

Chapter 11
Radiation Fibrosis Syndrome

Michael Stubblefield, Kathy Chou, and Nabela Enam

Introduction

Approximately 50% of all cancer patients receive radiation therapy (RT) during their disease course [1]. Radiation can be used as monotherapy (i.e., cervical cancers), as neoadjuvant or adjuvant therapy (i.e., breast cancer), or in combination with chemotherapy (i.e., head and neck cancer) [2]. Radiation treatment is the application of electromagnetic radiation (x-rays, gamma rays, electrons) to tissue. As these rays pass through cells, the ionizing energy damages DNA, releases free radicals, and subsequently signals for apoptosis when the cells undergo mitosis. There are several types of RT available including superficial x-rays (orthovoltage), brachytherapy, radio-isotopes, protons, and megavoltage radiotherapy [2]. The measure of radiation dose is the Gray (Gy); 1 gray is defined as 1 Joule of energy applied to 1 kg of tissue. Note that 1 Gy = 1000 cGy and is also commonly used to express radiation dosing.

When RT was being developed for clinical use, large and frequent doses were the mainstay of treatment. However, it

M. Stubblefield (✉) · K. Chou · N. Enam
Physical Medicine and Rehabilitation, Kessler Institute for Rehabilitation, West Orange, NJ, USA
e-mail: mstubblefield@selectmedical.com

© Springer Nature Switzerland AG 2020
J. Baima, A. Khanna (eds.), *Cancer Rehabilitation*,
https://doi.org/10.1007/978-3-030-44462-4_11

was found that patients suffered adverse reactions, generally in direct correlation with the total dose of radiation, size of each fraction, and size of the radiation field. Advances such as intensity-modulated radiotherapy and stereotactic radio-surgical techniques more precisely localize radiation to tumor cells while sparing the surrounding normal tissue. Despite advances in technique, normal tissue is often still involved in the radiation field and subject to damage. The side effects of radiation occur early (within days) or late (within years), and can affect any organ system. Skin and mucosa are predominantly affected in the acute phase. In the late phase, vascular damage and fibrosis are the primary reactions [2].

Radiation fibrosis (RF) is typically a delayed complication of radiation therapy and refers to the pathologic formation of fibrotic tissue over time. Risk factors include a patient's age, comorbidities, and concurrent oncologic treatment in addition to specific radiation factors, such as size of the radiation field, total dose, dose per fraction, type of tissue radiated, and the time from initial radiation treatment [3]. There are three histopathologic phases of RF: pre-fibrotic, fibrotic, and late fibro-atrophic. The first is often asymptomatic, and characterized by chronic local inflammation, increased permeability, and edema typically in the first few months following therapy. In the following organized fibrotic phase, patches of activated fibroblasts form a disorganized extracellular matrix interspersed with senescent fibroblasts. This sclerotic tissue can develop and progress several years after therapy. The final fibro-atrophic stage usually presents several years after therapy with dense and friable tissue [4, 5].

The clinical manifestations of RF are termed Radiation Fibrosis Syndrome (RFS). RFS can involve any tissue including any component of the central or peripheral nervous system within or traversing through the radiation field. The clinical manifestations include neuromuscular, musculoskeletal, and functional sequelae, as described below [3].

Complications

The complications of radiation-induced damage result from direct or indirect effects of progressive fibrotic sclerosis. Any body system can be affected including cardiovascular, pulmonary, endocrine, integumentary, gastrointestinal, etc. Damage to the neuromuscular and musculoskeletal systems can be profound and severely limit function and quality of life. Neuromuscular damage can affect the brain, spinal cord, nerve roots, plexus, peripheral nerves, and muscles. Identifying and naming the specific structures involved, for instance, "myelo-radiculo-plexo-neuro-myopathy," is important to clarify the underlying pathology and its relation to other functional issues [3]. Musculoskeletal pathology from radiation fibrosis results from bone, tendon, and ligament involvement. Overall, the management of clinical manifestations of radiation fibrosis is supportive as the fibrotic sclerosis underlying the syndrome is irreversible and will likely progress over time. The treatment and modalities primarily include therapy, medications, orthotics, and injections [6].

Progression of fibrotic sclerosis can affect the macro and microvasculature, leading to ischemia with resultant motor and sensory defects. Irritation to the spinothalamic tracts or damage to the somatosensory nervous system may cause central neuropathic (i.e., funicular) or peripheral neuropathic pain, respectively [6]. Nerve stabilizing medications such as gabapentin, pregabalin, and duloxetine are often effective for neuropathic pain associated with RFS. Second-line agents include tricyclic antidepressants. Nonsteroidal anti-inflammatory drugs and opiates may also provide some relief [6].

When only a single peripheral nerve is involved, the patient may present with deficits specific to that nerve. For example, an affected dorsal scapular nerve would result in rhomboid weakness, while suprascapular nerve involvement would show supraspinatus weakness, and spinal accessory nerve damage may manifest as trapezius dysfunction. Often, multiple peripheral nerves are involved. Inflammation, irritation, or compression at the level of the spinal nerve root or at the brachial or lumbosacral plexus could result in a radiculopathy or plexopathy, and may require electrodiagnostic studies for differentiation. When occurring at the level of the spinal cord, the outcome is myelopathy and if affecting muscle fibers, myopathy in the form of spasms or dystonia may result [6]. At the tendon and ligament level, radiation fibrosis reduces elasticity by causing shortening of structures and contracture formation. When bone is targeted, it can become brittle and more susceptible to injury and neoplasm development [6].

Clinical Syndromes and Management

As radiation fibrosis is progressive, patients exposed to radiation gradually develop symptoms, but the onset and clinical manifestations vary depending on an individual's risk factors and type of radiation exposure. Currently, there are no formal recommendations for treating RFS due to the multifaceted pathophysiology as well as difficulty in establishing outcome measures. Interventions are being evaluated to target the suspected pathophysiology of fibrosis, including anti-inflammatory agents, vascular therapy with hyperbaric oxygen, and antioxidant treatment [4]. To date, the mainstay of treatment is focused on symptomatic relief and removal of aggravating factors. Some of the most common presentations and their management are described below.

Neck extensor weakness, often termed "dropped head syndrome" is commonly seen and develops as a result of atrophy and weakness of the cervical and thoracic paraspinal muscles and shoulder girdle. The neuromuscular dysfunction leads to inability to elevate the head, poor posture, fatigue, and pain. Therapy primarily focuses on myofascial release of fibrotic structures to improve posture, postural retraining, neuromuscular re-education and strengthening, and restoring range of motion [3]. Cervical orthotics and local anesthetic injections can be useful for painful muscle spasms [5].

Shoulder pain and dysfunction occur when radiation targets the shoulder muscles directly or nerves innervating these structures. The rotator cuff musculature may become weakened thereby, affecting range of motion, causing protracted shoulders and misalignment of tendons leading to impingement that could progress to tendonitis or adhesive capsulitis [5]. In addition to symptomatic management with medications and injections, therapy emphasizing myofascial release, posture training, core and neck extensor and rotator cuff strengthening, and shoulder range of motion should be implemented.

Head and neck cancer patients treated with radiation to the neck can develop contractures of the anterior musculature including sternocleidomastoid, scalene, and trapezius muscles. This is often associated with painful muscle spasms, fatigue, and/or damage to the nerve roots, cervical plexus, and other nerves within the radiation field. Abnormal posture with or without loss of range of motion (cervical dystonia) often develops. The progressive hardening of neck musculature, tendons, and ligaments may interfere with swallowing, phonation, and other activities of daily living. These patients benefit from aggressive physical therapy to restore cervical mobility. Botulinum toxin used in conjunction with therapy can relieve muscle spasm and pain, but should generally only be done in the anterior neck to minimize the chance of precipitating or worsening neck extension weakness [3].

Trismus is impaired mouth opening, and typically occurs after radiation exposure to the head and neck. Fibrosis of the pterygoid and masseter muscles can cause spasms that affect oral hygiene, feeding, chewing, and swallowing. Physical therapy to improve mandibular range of motion is the first line of treatment. Botulinum toxin has been studied to improve pain and may consequently improve mouth movement. Dynamic jaw-opening devices have been shown to be effective in gradually increasing range of motion, and can also be used with therapeutic exercises to improve quality of life [3].

Clinical Cases

Case 1

A 49-year-old male with a history of human papilloma virus (HPV)-associated tonsil and throat cancer treated with combined chemoradiation developed neck pain and spasms with involvement of his left shoulder several years following his initial radiation treatment. His physical exam was notable for decreased range of motion with circumferential atrophy of the neck and tenderness to palpation most pronounced in the left sternocleidomastoid (SCM) and scalene muscles. Additionally, he had brisk reflexes and clonus in his left lower extremity, weakness in his deltoid and biceps muscles, and atrophy of his trapezius muscles as well as diffuse atrophy along the sites of radiation field exposure. Taken together, his clinical picture was consistent with radiation-induced myelo-radiculo-plexo-neuro-myopathy. Subsequent electrodiagnostic testing supported this diagnosis.

A trial of acupuncture and medical management with pregabalin gave no relief, while physical therapy and massage offered some benefit. The patient's primary concern was his impaired quality of life from the painful neck spasms consistent with cervical dystonia, which developed secondary to underlying neuromuscular damage from radiation. He received botulinum toxin type-A (Botox®) injections to his left SCM and scalene muscles with considerable relief, lasting approximately 2–3 months. During his follow-up evaluation, the decision was made to repeat botulinum toxin injections every 3 months with possible dose adjustments in addition to concurrent physical therapy and regular home exercise program.

Case 2

A 50-year-old female was diagnosed in her early 30s with stage IIB nodular sclerosing Hodgkin lymphoma involving her neck, mediastinum, and left hilum. She underwent chemoradiation therapy, but had multiple episodes of recurrence, which prompted further treatment with chemotherapy, radiation therapy, and stem cell transplantation for several more years. After extensive radiation exposure, she developed severe radiation fibrosis impacting her quality of life with respect to dressing, cooking, and toileting. Additionally, her impairments with activities of daily living progressively worsened over time. On exam, she was noted to have atrophy of her cervicothoracic musculature, right shoulder subluxation, decreased pulses in her left upper limb, and diminished sensation along her entire left upper limb, but also medial aspect of her right upper limb.

The patient's clinical picture was consistent with radiation-induced myelo-radiculo-plexo-neuro-myopathy, with significant bilateral brachial plexopathy and neck extensor weakness causing dropped head syndrome. The patient was prescribed physical and occupational therapy for myofascial release, core strengthening, postural retaining, and neuromuscular reeducation. She was also provided with a cervical collar as instructed on the importance of compliance with her home exercise program.

Case 3

A 51-year-old man with a history of diffuse large B-cell lymphoma diagnosed in 2006 was treated with chemotherapy and radiation to a large mediastinal tumor. He presented 13 years later with a 1-year history of severe left chest and back pain. The pain was described as radiating from his upper back around his left rib cage to the anterior midclavicular line. Medical management by his oncologist and primary care physician included epidural steroid injections, which offered some relief. He was also prescribed pharmacotherapy with varying doses of gabapentin, pregabalin, duloxetine, and opiates, which provided minimal relief.

On physical examination, he was found to have significant midline and paramedian atrophy of the pectoralis muscles, consistent with his radiation field exposure (Fig. 11.1). His neurologic exam was symmetric, with mild weakness in the proximal upper extremities but intact strength distally and in the bilateral lower extremities. He had no evidence of allodynia or hyperreflexia on exam, and his gait was normal. Magnetic Resonance Imaging (MRI) of his thoracic spine demonstrated a 4.1 cm ascending and proximal descending aortic aneurysm, multilevel thoracic degenerative disease with small disc herniations at T2-T3 and T11-T12 without cord or root compression, and fat replacement of the bone marrow in T1-T6 vertebrae, consistent with his history of radiation therapy (Fig. 11.2).

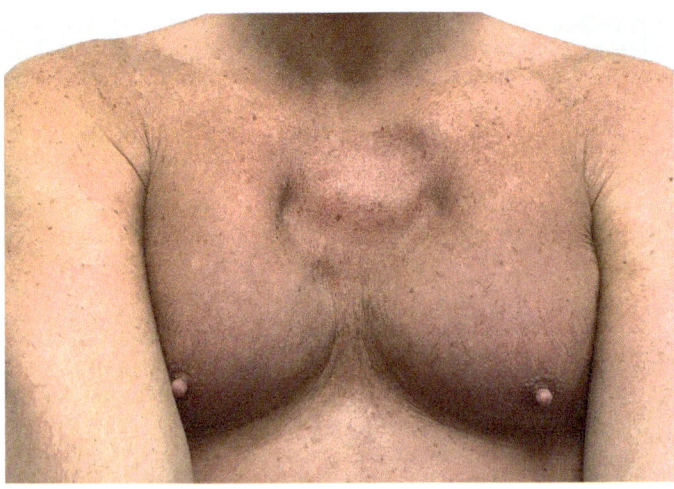

FIGURE 11.1 51-year-old male with significant radiation fibrosis of the medial pectoralis muscles after receiving radiation treatment for his large mediastinal lymphoma

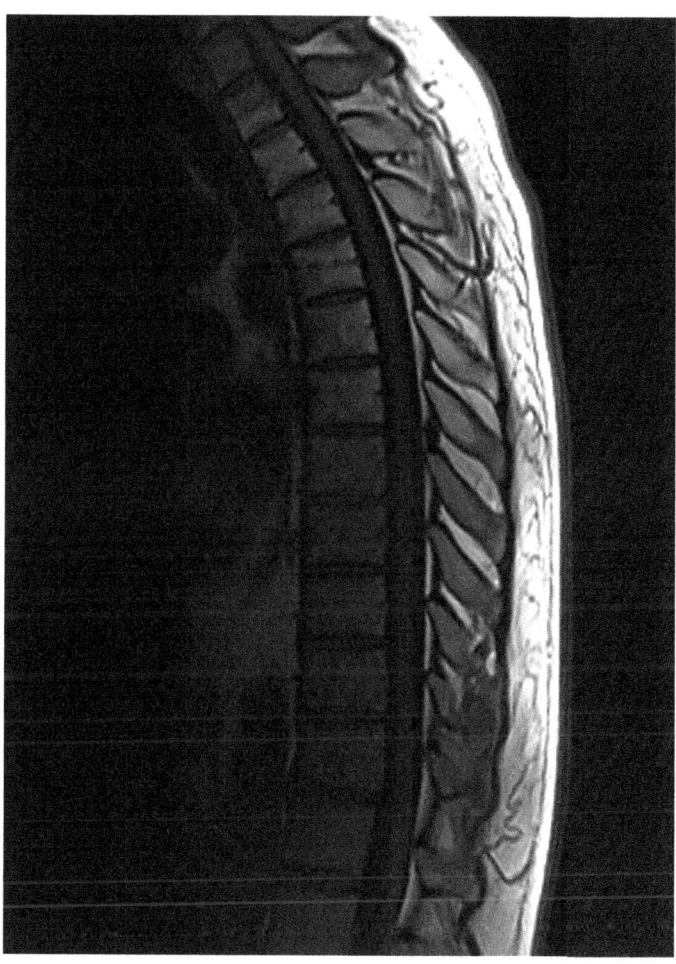

FIGURE 11.2 T1-weighted MRI without contrast of thoracic spine in patient with history of lymphoma treated with radiation showing multi-level thoracic degenerative disease. T1-T6 vertebral bodies demonstrate hyperintensity highly suggestive of fat replacement in bone marrow, likely due to radiation therapy

His findings were suggestive of radiation fibrosis causing thoracic radiculopathy with possible concurrent proximal intercostal mononeuropathies given that his radiation field included the upper thoracic spine and ascending and descending aorta. The patient was amenable to a re-trial of neuropathic agents starting with gradual up-titration of pregabalin in addition to adjunctive medications as needed.

Multiple Choice Questions

1. Radiation fibrosis may affect which of the following:

   A. Heart
   B. Vasculature
   C. Muscles
   D. B and C
   E. All of the above

2. A 52-year-old female with a history of Hodgkin lymphoma at age 24 was treated with mantle radiation. Three years ago she was diagnosed with right breast cancer treated with mastectomy, chemotherapy, and radiation to the breast and chest wall. She presents with progressive right upper extremity weakness affecting the deltoid, biceps, triceps, and entire hand. Damage to which structure is likely the major cause of her weakness?

   A. Cervical nerve roots
   B. Cervical plexus
   C. Brachial plexus
   D. Axillary nerve
   E. Median nerve

3. A 46-year-old male with squamous cell carcinoma of the oral cavity was treated with surgical resection and combined chemotherapy and radiation therapy completing 1 year ago. He presents with jaw pain and difficulty opening his mouth. His median interincisal opening is 15 mm. In addition to physical therapy, what is the next best adjunctive therapy to consider for his treatment?

A. Surgery
B. Botulinum toxin injection
C. Jaw-opening device
D. A and B
E. B and C

4. A 61-year-old female with a history of hypertension and Hodgkin's Lymphoma of the mediastinum is treated with MOPP chemotherapy and mantle radiation 31 years ago presents to clinic complaining of progressive difficulty performing household tasks, particularly when raising her right arm above shoulder level. Physical exam reveals positive Neer's and Hawkin's tests, consistent with shoulder impingement. Radiation effects on which structure are most likely contributing significantly to her symptoms?

A. Cerebellum
B. Spinal cord
C. Cervical plexus
D. Cervical nerve roots
E. Phrenic nerve

5. Which of the following is NOT true of radiation fibrosis?

A. Any part of the central or peripheral nervous system within the radiation field can be involved
B. Opiates and tricyclic antidepressants may offer some benefit in treating symptoms
C. Following radiation therapy, patients in the initial stage of radiation fibrosis may be asymptomatic
D. With appropriate management, radiation fibrosis may be reversible
E. Bones, tendons, and ligaments can be affected

Answers

1. E
2. C
3. E
4. D
5. D

References

1. Jaffray DA, Gospodarowicz MK. Radiation therapy for cancer. In: Gelband H, et al., editors. Cancer: disease control priorities, vol. 3. 3rd ed. Washington, DC: The International Bank for Reconstruction and Development / The World Bank; 2015.
2. Thankamma Ajithkumar HH, Cook N. Concepts of multidisciplinary management. In: Oncology (Oxford desk reference). New York: Oxford University Press; 2011.
3. Stubblefield MD. Radiation fibrosis syndrome: neuromuscular and musculoskeletal complications in cancer survivors. PM R. 2011;3(11):1041–54.
4. Delanian S, Lefaix JL. The radiation-induced fibroatrophic process: therapeutic perspective via the antioxidant pathway. Radiother Oncol. 2004;73(2):119–31.
5. Stubblefield MD. Clinical evaluation and management of radiation fibrosis syndrome. Phys Med Rehabil Clin N Am. 2017;28(1):89–100.
6. Stubblefield MD. Neuromuscular complications of radiation therapy. Muscle Nerve. 2017;56(6):1031–40.

Chapter 12
Conclusion: Innovative Research

Andrea Cheville

Introduction

A convergence of economic, technological, policy, and scientific forces are driving changes in the nature and scope of cancer rehabilitation services, who receives and provides them, and where they are provided. Researchers have both fueled and reacted to these changes, and in so doing contributed new knowledge that will shape how the clinical community responds to continued advances. The last decade has witnessed a striking shift away from use of conventional antineoplastic therapies to the adoption of a new arsenal of biological agents that offer unprecedented effectiveness in some contexts. In parallel, marked demographic expansion of older, more medically and functionally morbid cancer patients has catalyzed growth in geriatric oncology and placed increasing downstream pressure on caregivers who manage toxicity and morbidity among this vulnerable population. Oncology care providers are also responding to observations by the National Academy of Medicine (NAM), Centers for Disease Control and Prevention, National Cancer Institute, and National Quality Forum (NQF), among other influential bod-

A. Cheville (✉)
Department of Physical Medicine and Rehabilitation, Mayo Clinic, Rochester, MN, USA
e-mail: Cheville.Andrea@mayo.edu

© Springer Nature Switzerland AG 2020   169
J. Baima, A. Khanna (eds.), *Cancer Rehabilitation*,
https://doi.org/10.1007/978-3-030-44462-4_12

ies, that care experiences and Quality of Life among patients with cancer, despite the staggering out-of-pocket costs they bear, leave much to be desired [1].

These changes represent the tip of the iceberg. Enumeration of ongoing and anticipated changes in the factors that will shape cancer rehabilitation's content and delivery is an exhaustive and, ultimately, speculative prospect. This chapter attempts to highlight changes that are already underway, based on a strong evidentiary foundation.

Models of Cancer Rehabilitation Service Delivery

Background Fee-for-service (FFS) reimbursement has dominated clinical payment for decades despite efforts, most notably Health Maintenance Organizations, to establish credible alternatives. Care delivery has been profoundly shaped by the point-of-care, clinic-based contact required by most fee-for-service reimbursement. This requirement has persisted despite recognition that face-to-face encounters are inconvenient and costly for many patients, limit access, and are frequently unnecessary. Fee-for-service has also constrained care delivery for clinical contacts devoted to monitoring, education, and support.

Several trends have conspired to challenge the dominance of fee-for-service; most salient among these is an increasing recognition that paying for inappropriate, low value, and ineffective care does not advance patient or national interests. Empowered, tech savvy healthcare consumers are demanding improved convenience and experience. Influential organizations such as the NQF and NAM, as well as payers, have highlighted compensation informed by patient-reported outcomes and experience as essential to improvement in the US healthcare system [2]. That patients' perspectives, as systematically assessed with process and outcome measures, should be a driving force in shaping our healthcare system has advanced value-based reimbursement, and was a defining feature of the Patient Protection and Affordable Care Act.

The possibilities for cancer rehabilitation service provision created by shifts away from fee-for-service are profound. They open the door to a radical reconceptualization of healthcare delivery, and create a pressing need for evidence to inform strategies to render care delivery more patient-centric while simultaneously preserving effectiveness and enhancing value. Unquestionably some healthcare services yield best results when delivered in accordance with FFS mandates; however, in many cases we lack knowledge to distinguish these, or to identify components of complex multi-step care delivery processes that could be provided remotely. This lack is particularly troublesome for rehabilitation medicine as our goal is to enhance patients' function and comfort outside of clinical settings in the communities and homes. However, the potential for striking advances is also great since shifts away from FFS offer an opportunity to leverage the burgeoning IT capabilities to remotely assess, prompt, coach, educate, and direct patients as they engage in their "real world" lives.

The fact that patients with cancer prioritize their autonomy and ability to function should further potentiate the expansion of cancer rehabilitation service delivery models beyond the constraints of FFS. Additionally, patients' functional status is associated with key outcomes: survival, return to work, and healthcare utilization [3, 4]. Therefore, care that preserves and enhances patients' function is integral to value-based purchasing initiatives. With the relaxing of FFS' reimbursement requirement for center-based delivery, many options become viable that may ultimately prove far better matched to patients' needs for the behavioral changes and activity enhancement required for enduring functional preservations.

Cutting edge Remote and hybrid (combination remote-center based) approaches have been validated that evaluate, educate, and treat patients with cancer to address diverse clinical targets. For example, two randomized controlled trials that provided collaborative telecare via phone calls and web-based interfaces noted clinically meaningfully benefits and were cost effective. The INCPAD trial addressed pain and depression [5, 6], while the COPE trial addressed functional decline [7]. Further strides have been made in the ease, precision, and cost of remote patient assessments, spurring broader clinical integration. Patient-reported outcome (PRO)-based measures are being leveraged to make determinations of when and which rehabilitation services should be initiated [8, 9]. Additionally, through electronic health records (EHR)-based and other electronic platforms, PRO responses can trigger branching logic allowing for highly individualized assessments.

Objective patient data has also become easier to capture remotely. The feasibility of monitoring patients' function using sensors and life space-based approaches has become progressively cheaper and more precise with smaller more responsive devices. Data from wearable monitors can be uploaded into current generation EHRs from graphical display to patients and clinicians, allowing associations to be made between behavioral, clinical, and physiological parameters. Use of these data allows clinicians to base their decision-making on accurate, higher-volume information than has been previously available. In addition, clinicians now have the capacity to remotely suggest small, nuanced changes to a patient's regimen based on these data without requiring a clinic visit. Patients can be tracked, and small but meaningful changes detected to inform treatment without the costly and burdensome requirement for repeated clinician evaluations.

Remote education has become well established in academia, and is gaining clinical traction. Diverse formats are currently in clinical use: synchronous (real-time) and asynchronous (delayed) one-to-one and one-to-many, as well as interactive and one-way didactic formats. The platforms that have been used to support these exchanges are equally diverse: IT chat groups, video conferencing, email list serves, and teleconferencing, many for cancer-related education. Reports of improved patient engagement, activation, and outcomes with remote educational initiatives suggest that use of these platforms will increase [10, 11].

Future The expansion of validated remote delivery models has been principally constrained by reimbursement. As more liberal, value-based payments that focus on outcomes gain traction, the potential to provide patients with function-oriented care when and how they need it will inevitably grow. Current federally pragmatic trials are evaluating models that strive to match the symptom and function needs of cancer patients with preference-matched, readily accessible care that encourages timely care team engagement and self-management. Systematically collecting PROs and either reporting these data to patients' care teams or using the data to trigger EHR-based clinical decision support to manage symptoms and disablement in a proactive rather than reactive manner, may improve utilization, clinical and patient-reported outcomes.

These interventions will formally evaluate remote treatment approaches that are being steadily integrated in cancer care. As has been the case for other advances, the industry's appetite for innovation will not wait on evidence. Consequently, remote care delivery approaches are steadily making their way into clinical practice, and many clinicians are organically incorporating these into patient management. It is therefore reasonable to anticipate that anecdotal reports, as well as those from hypothesis-driven research, will shape the future.

Big Data, Artificial Intelligence, and Electronic Health Records

"Big data," or population-level aggregated data collected in the course of care delivery and billing, has held the attention of clinical researchers for over a decade and that interest and related expectations have intensified [12]. In part, this increased focus has been driven by the availability of data sets representing large sectors of the US population, >100 million patients, that include granular clinical, treatment, and demographic information. These data allow researchers to ask questions that are not feasible in clinical trials and would be cripplingly expensive as cohort studies regarding long-term outcomes and treatment effectiveness in important but difficult-to-access patient subgroups.

Interest has been piqued to an even greater extent by the potential for applying artificial, or augmented, intelligence (AI) to these datasets and developing algorithms to directly influence care through electronic health records (EHRs) and other media [13, 14]. The concept of such "knowledge creation" by integrating clinical data of staggering breadth with respect to both volume and type, has already been operationalized in EHR-based "sniffers" that identify patients with incipient sepsis, impending ICU transfer, and palliative care needs [15]. These examples all highlight the fact that subtle signals indicating a need for immediate or near-term change in management can be buried in a sea of competing signals and fall below critical thresholds for recognition by human awareness.

While "big data" approaches to characterizing shifting needs in rehabilitation medicine have yielded insights, AI and EHR-based applications have been more limited. For example, by examining administrative claims data, Ottenbacher et al. described steadily increasing admission rates of patients to inpatient rehabilitation facilities (IRFs) with debility diagnoses, often due to cancer, in lieu of more conventional rehabilitation diagnoses, associated with a higher rate of acute care readmissions in this subgroup [16]. As of yet, insights from PMR "big data" efforts have illustrated such prevailing trends, rather than yielding pragmatic targets for intervention.

Cutting edge Ongoing efforts in fields outside of PMR are examining whether and how the promise of AI will be realized. Some of these conform to conventional research methods, while others are conducted by providers and investors to create potentially lucrative intellectual property (IP). One lesson has become clear, it is insufficient to simply present yet another value, e.g., risk estimate, via EHRs without tactical implementation that enables clinical end users to appropriately assimilate and respond to the information. Consequently, implementation science has become an increasing focus of national funding initiatives. EHR usability studies are similarly ongoing and insights can be anticipated in coming years.

Current efforts to systematically collect functional and rehabilitation-related outcome data through the EHR will likely fuel future AI-based approaches. In many ways PMR outcomes are an ideal target for AI since AI approaches work well when predicting binary (Yes/No) outcomes, e.g., the patient did/did not require post acute care, return to work, get readmitted, fall, etc. [17]. With the collection of function PROs in routine clinical care, the range of outcomes that may be predicted through AI will expand.

Our ability to operationally leverage AI-derived estimates of risk, response, and other clinical vital parameters to inform decision-making is also advancing precipitously with the increasing sophistication of EHR-based clinical decision support (CDS) tools. CDS refers to a broad range of EHR functionality designed to help clinicians respond rapidly and appropriately to clinical data through alerts, preconfigured orders, data presentation (graphs, tables, text), prompts, among many other approaches [18]. Although few reports, as yet, have described the application of CDS approaches to rehabilitation service delivery, this will likely change given success documented in other clinical areas. For example, by combining PRO-based screening for current smoking and interest in quitting with information provided directly to patients regarding local cessation programs and alerts/prompts to physicians to place preconfigured program referral orders, one institution increased program referrals tenfold [19]. CDS tools that directly push information to patient portals are gaining traction and offer unprecedented opportunities to address behavioral determinants of health, including exercise and physical inactivity. Also, the potential to introduce patients to relatively simple function-directed interventions via their portals offers the possibility to deliver stepped care as endorsed by current models of cancer rehabilitation that match incrementally intense care with patient need and complexity [20].

Future As researchers and industry create the building blocks for the AI-directed individualization of health care, novel approaches will inevitably follow and likely impact cancer rehabilitation service delivery. AI algorithms imbedded in EHRs can automatically abstract clinical data in real time and update patients risk and outcome predictions on a dynamic, ongoing basis. The ground is fertile, as mentioned above, for AI to anticipate and thereby tactically direct care to enhance cancer rehabilitation outcomes in an individualized manner.

"Precision" Impairment Management

The use of enhanced imaging strategies, genomics, and biomarkers to direct less-invasive "precision medicine" treatments for disease processes has been a focus of intensive investigation, become established in other specialties, and gained steady traction for impairment management in rehabilitation medicine [21]. For example, the use of ultrasound guidance for minimally invasive carpal tunnel release is slowly displacing open surgical release. The research and clinical advances that permit such paradigmatic shifts in management are, for the most part, steadily incremental. However, they seem to have reached a critical mass such that major shifts in established management approaches have become a regular occurrence. The revolution in biological cancer therapies is a salient example. Elegant, individualized targeting of tumors based on DNA profiling is now the accepted standard of care.

While precision medicine has yet to become a potent influence on cancer rehabilitation practice, gradual shifts and small advances suggest that its feasibility may abruptly change as occurred in medical oncology. Further, advances in certain lines of preclinical inquiry, e.g., aerobic conditioning to regulate intra-tumoral vascular maturity and perfusion, hypoxia, and metabolism, suggest that the current dichotomy between treatments targeting neoplasia and physical impairments may blur and ultimately break down [22]. An optimally individualized, precision approach may comprehensively consider a patient's cancer, comorbidities, impairments, and predisposition to specific toxicities in order to simultaneously maximize outcomes across multiple critical domains rather than the relative narrow and condition-specific outcomes that currently dominate.

Cutting edge There are several areas relevant to cancer rehabilitation in which precision approaches have shown promise. Lee Jones et al., have blazed a novel trail in demonstrating that exercise may be prescribed with granular precision to potentially mediate changes in tumor cell mitochondrial metabolism and composition of the tumor microenvironment [23, 24]. Kathryn Schmitz et al. have similarly studied biomarkers associated with different types of exercise to develop individualized programs that not only reduce risk of cancer recurrence, but also enhance patients' functional abilities [25, 26].

Lymphedema has been a focus of several important recent innovations that have the potential to yield pragmatic precision medicine approaches. The use of indocyanine green (ICG) mapping of distal lymphatics to identify collateral drainage pathways, as well as sites for surgical lympho-venous bypass grafting, has established precedent for novel means to individualize treatments by applying heretofore unavailable insights into patient-level variation. A trial is currently underway comparing lymphedema management that includes ICG-imaging-directed manual lymphatic drainage versus standard drainage, which varies minimally across patients. ICG imaging has also been proposed as a means of more precisely staging lymphedema and capturing the known variations in stage within an affected body part that have, to this point, remained largely indistinguishable [27], as well as to identify anomalous and dysfunctional lymphatic channels for ablation [28].

Additional work in lymphedema has characterized the exact inflammatory mediators that drive the progressive fibrosis responsible for the condition's characteristic worsening over time. Stan Rockson et al. identified leukotriene LTB_4 as a critical target for blocking inflammation-related lymphedematous progression [29]. This work led to recently reported trials testing ketoprofen inhibition of leukotriene LTB_4 that noted significantly reductions in the dermal metaplasia that distinguishes Stage II from III lymphedema [30]. The potential import of this finding cannot be overstated as it is the first successful mechanistically targeted approach to curbing lymphedema's inexorable progression with the potential to reduce onerous and quality-of-life-degrading requirements for manual therapy.

Future The intensity of current investigative efforts devoted to genomic- and biomarker-based prediction of treatment response and toxicity ensures that precision oncology will become an increasingly established standard of care. Emergent imaging approaches that obviate the requirement for pathological confirmation of some cancer types, as well as the application of AI algorithms to image interpretation for optimized treatment selection, are further examples of current investigative approaches that are expected to yield near-term clinical applications. As functional outcomes are more systematically captured in oncologic care, there will be expanding opportunities to rigorously characterize the degree to which the diverse data sources that fuel precision oncology can be concurrently leveraged to predict functional outcomes and direct cancer rehabilitation service delivery. Additionally, the growing sophistication of ultrasound-directed minimally invasive musculoskeletal treatments and regenerative rehabilitation approaches, particularly those using stem cells to promote tissue repair, offer promising opportunities for "precision cancer rehabilitation."

Nonpharmacological Pain Management

The opioid epidemic has forever changed the public's awareness of pain prevalence, the limitations of current pain management approaches, and the formidable harms associated with unchecked use of habit-forming drugs. Not surprisingly, even though cancer has remained a "carve out" among guidelines promulgated by federal and specialty organizations that recommend aggressive restraint in opioid prescribing, alarm has grown over the high rates of persistent opioid use among disease-free cancer survivors [31, 32].

A large federal investment in research to catalyze innovation in the management of pain and opioid use disorder has already yielded novel insights. However, it has also highlighted the need for integrated care delivery approaches that address the psychosocial underpinnings of persistent and unresponsive pain. This need is no less acute among cancer populations than it is for the general public. In fact, an argument has been made that in some contexts it is more so since dependency-inducing, centrally acting medications, e.g., opioids and benzodiazepines, are liberally prescribed to patients with cancer even though at least half of the patients will experience persistent psychosocial stressors which have the potential to mediate aberrant and prolonged substance use [33].

Multimodal pain management with an emphasis on nonpharmacological approaches has therefore become a renewed topic of investigative attention. While lacking the novelty of "precision medicine," efforts to address the knowledge gap regarding how to expediently identify which therapies may benefit specific patients and how to ensure patients' access to high fidelity treatments is no less critical. Given the scope of the problem and the requirement to deliver therapies at scale, it is not surprising that interest has turned to telecare approaches. However, many of the patient subgroups at risk for poor outcomes lack the IT resources.

Cutting edge In addition to new analgesic molecule and device development, current research efforts are developing new approaches to care delivery that may prove highly relevant to cancer rehabilitation. The use of health coaches to support patients in setting individually relevant goals related to coping effectively with pain and anxiety, as well as recovering functional abilities, has proven effective, as well as cost effective in some populations [34–36]. A number of studies are currently examining multimodal approaches that use the EHR to identify patients with intense and persistent pain, and connect them with coaches and other support services. Thus far rehabilitation providers have featured limitedly in these efforts.

Research efforts to apply novel electromagnetic therapies to cancer rehabilitation populations are also ongoing. Recently, Scrambler therapy® has emerged as a benign and potentially effective treatment for CIPN and other cancer-associated neuropathic pain states [37]. Although several case series reported benefit from the application of Scrambler therapy treatments to cancer pain syndromes [38, 39], a trial involving patients with chemotherapy-induced peripheral neuropathy was negative [40]. Nonetheless, promising results have spurred investigators to seek funding for electromedical pain management therapy trials to address other cancer pain syndromes.

Future Undoubtedly, novel pain treatment will emerge from the flurry of research activity incited by funding priorities. Cancer rehabilitation physicians will likely learn of the anticipated new drugs and devices through conventional means. However, of perhaps greater relevance to cancer rehabilitation will be the novel models of multimodal pain management that are being developed and validated. However, these will require more concerted effort to learn of and apply the findings.

Conclusion

Forecasting is challenging, yet it is safe to conclude that the research trends described above will create opportunities to expand and enhance the scope and effectiveness of cancer rehabilitation. These trends will undoubtedly cross-fertilize and inform each other over time in response to the mounting demand to improve health care value and patient experience.

References

1. National Academies of Sciences, Engineering, and Medicine. Long-term survivorship care after cancer treatment: proceedings of a workshop. Washington, DC: The National Academies Press. 2018.
2. Forum NQ. Patient reported outcomes (PROs) in performance measurement. Washington, DC: The National Quality Forum. 2013.
3. Quality AfHRa. Total expenses and percent distribution for selected conditions by type of service: United States, 2014. Medical Expenditure Panel Survey Household Component Data. 3 Aug 2017 ed 2016.
4. Lage DE, Nipp RD, D'Arpino SM, et al. Predictors of posthospital transitions of care in patients with advanced cancer. J Clin Oncol. 2018;36:76–82.
5. Choi Yoo SJ, Nyman JA, Cheville AL, Kroenke K. Cost effectiveness of telecare management for pain and depression in patients with cancer: results from a randomized trial. Gen Hosp Psychiatry. 2014;36:599–606.
6. Kroenke K, Theobald D, Wu J, et al. Effect of telecare management on pain and depression in patients with cancer: a randomized trial. JAMA. 2010;304:163–71.
7. Cheville AL, Moynihan T, Herrin J, Loprinzi C, Kroenke K. Effect of collaborative telerehabilitation on functional impairment and pain among patients with advanced-stage cancer: a randomized clinical trial. JAMA Oncol. 2019;5(5):644–52.

8. Cella D, Choi S, Garcia S, et al. Setting standards for severity of common symptoms in oncology using the PROMIS item banks and expert judgment. Qual Life Res. 2014;23:2651–61.

9. Cella D, Choi S, Rosenbloom S, et al. A novel IRT-based case-ranking approach to derive expert standards for symptom severity. Qual Life Res. 2008;17:A–32.

10. Galiano-Castillo N, Cantarero-Villanueva I, Fernandez-Lao C, et al. Telehealth system: a randomized controlled trial evaluating the impact of an internet-based exercise intervention on quality of life, pain, muscle strength, and fatigue in breast cancer survivors. Cancer. 2016;122:3166–74.

11. Atema V, van Leeuwen M, Kieffer JM, et al. Efficacy of internet-based cognitive behavioral therapy for treatment-induced menopausal symptoms in breast cancer survivors: results of a randomized controlled trial. J Clin Oncol. 2019;37:809–22.

12. Shah ND, Steyerberg EW, Kent DM. Big data and predictive analytics: recalibrating expectations. JAMA. 2018;320:27–8.

13. Afzal M, Hussain M, Ali Khan W, et al. Comprehensible knowledge model creation for cancer treatment decision making. Comput Biol Med. 2017;82:119–29.

14. Yu P, Artz D, Warner J. Electronic health records (EHRs): supporting ASCO's vision of cancer care. Am Soc Clin Oncol Educ Book. 2014;1:225–31.

15. Herasevich V, Afessa B, Chute CG, Gajic O. Designing and testing computer based screening engine for severe sepsis/septic shock. AMIA Annu Symp Proc. 2008;1:966.

16. Galloway RV, Karmarkar AM, Graham JE, et al. Hospital readmission following discharge from inpatient rehabilitation for older adults with debility. Phys Ther. 2016;96:241–51.

17. Park SH, Han K. Methodologic guide for evaluating clinical performance and effect of artificial intelligence technology for medical diagnosis and prediction. Radiology. 2018;286:800–9.

18. Wright A, Sittig DF, Ash JS, Sharma S, Pang JE, Middleton B. Clinical decision support capabilities of commercially-available clinical information systems. J Am Med Inform Assoc. 2009;16:637–44.

19. Miner D. Building clinical programs around patient-entered data. Epic Users Group Meeting; Verona, WI; 2016.

20. Cheville AL, Mustian K, Winters-Stone K, Zucker DS, Gamble GL, Alfano CM. Cancer rehabilitation: an overview of current need, delivery models, and levels of care. Phys Med Rehabil Clin N Am. 2017;28:1–17.

21. Collins FS, Varmus H. A new initiative on precision medicine. N Engl J Med. 2015;372:793–5.
22. Ashcraft KA, Warner AB, Jones LW, Dewhirst MW. Exercise as adjunct therapy in cancer. Semin Radiat Oncol. 2019;29:16–24.
23. Lu M, Sanderson SM, Zessin A, et al. Exercise inhibits tumor growth and central carbon metabolism in patient-derived xenograft models of colorectal cancer. Cancer Metab. 2018;6:14.
24. Koelwyn GJ, Quail DF, Zhang X, White RM, Jones LW. Exercise-dependent regulation of the tumour microenvironment. Nat Rev Cancer. 2017;17:620–32.
25. Schmitz KH, Williams NI, Kontos D, et al. Dose-response effects of aerobic exercise on estrogen among women at high risk for breast cancer: a randomized controlled trial. Breast Cancer Res Treat. 2015;154:309–18.
26. Brown JC, Troxel AB, Ky B, et al. Dose-response effects of aerobic exercise among colon cancer survivors: a randomized phase II trial. Clin Colorectal Cancer. 2018;17:32–40.
27. Yamamoto T, Yamamoto N, Doi K, et al. Indocyanine green-enhanced lymphography for upper extremity lymphedema: a novel severity staging system using dermal backflow patterns. Plast Reconstr Surg. 2011;128:941–7.
28. Hara H, Mihara M. Indocyanine green lymphographic and lymphoscintigraphic findings in genital lymphedema-genital pathway score. Lymphat Res Biol. 2017;15:356–9.
29. Jiang X, Nicolls MR, Tian W, Rockson SG. Lymphatic dysfunction, leukotrienes, and lymphedema. Annu Rev Physiol. 2018;80:49–70.
30. Rockson SG, Tian W, Jiang X, et al. Pilot studies demonstrate the potential benefits of antiinflammatory therapy in human lymphedema. JCI Insight. 2018;3:20.
31. Fredheim OM, Skurtveit S, Handal M, Hjellvik V. A complete national cohort study of prescriptions of analgesics and benzodiazepines to cancer survivors in Norway 10 years after diagnosis. Pain. 2019;160:852–9.
32. Salz T, Lavery JA, Lipitz-Snyderman AN, et al. Trends in opioid use among older survivors of colorectal, lung, and breast cancers. J Clin Oncol. 2019;37:1001–11.
33. Barbera L, Sutradhar R, Howell D, et al. Factors associated with opioid use in long-term cancer survivors. J Pain Symptom Manag. 2019;58(1):100–107.e2.
34. Matthias MS, Daggy J, Adams J, et al. Evaluation of a peer coach-led intervention to improve pain symptoms (ECLIPSE): ratio-

nale, study design, methods, and sample characteristics. Contemp Clin Trials. 2019;81:71–9.

35. Benzo RP, Kramer KM, Hoult JP, Anderson PM, Begue IM, Seifert SJ. Development and feasibility of a home pulmonary rehabilitation program with health coaching. Respir Care. 2018;63:131–40.

36. Benzo RP, Kirsch JL, Hathaway JC, McEvoy CE, Vickers KS. Health coaching in severe COPD after a hospitalization: a qualitative analysis of a large randomized study. Respir Care. 2017;62:1403–11.

37. Marineo G, Iorno V, Gandini C, Moschini V, Smith TJ. Scrambler therapy may relieve chronic neuropathic pain more effectively than guideline-based drug management: results of a pilot, randomized, controlled trial. J Pain Symptom Manag. 2012;43:87–95.

38. Smith T, Cheville AL, Loprinzi CL, Longo-Schoberlein D. Scrambler therapy for the treatment of chronic post-mastectomy pain (cPMP). Cureus. 2017;9:e1378.

39. Pachman DR, Weisbrod BL, Seisler DK, et al. Pilot evaluation of Scrambler therapy for the treatment of chemotherapy-induced peripheral neuropathy. Support Care Cancer. 2015;23:943–51.

40. Smith TJ, Razzak AR, Blackford AL, et al. A pilot randomized sham-controlled trial of MC5-A scrambler therapy in the treatment of chronic chemotherapy-induced peripheral neuropathy (CIPN). J Palliat Care. 2019;35(1):53–8. https://doi.org/10.1177/825859719827589.

Index

© Springer Nature Switzerland AG 2020
J. Baima, A. Khanna (eds.), *Cancer Rehabilitation*,
https://doi.org/10.1007/978-3-030-44462-4

The manufacturer's authorised representative in the EU is Springer
Nature Customer Service Centre GmbH, Europaplatz 3, 69115 Heidelberg,
Germany. If you have any concerns regarding our products, please
contact ProductSafety@springernature.com

Printed and bound by CPI Group (UK) Ltd, Croydon, CR0 4YY
24/04/2026
02096309-0001